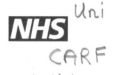

UCL Hospitals Injectable
Medicines Administration Guide

Second Edition

Pharmacy Department
University College London Hospitals

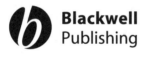 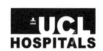

Blackwell Publishing   **UCL HOSPITALS**

© 1998, 2007 Pharmacy Department, University College London Hospitals

Blackwell Publishing editorial offices:
Blackwell Publishing Ltd, 9600 Garsington Road, Oxford OX4 2DQ, UK
Tel: +44 (0)1865 776868
Blackwell Publishing Inc., 350 Main Street, Malden, MA 02148–5020, USA
Tel: +1 781 388 8250
Blackwell Publishing Asia Pty Ltd, 550 Swanston Street, Carlton, Victoria 3053,
Australia
Tel: +61 (0)3 8359 1011

First published 1998
Second edition published 2007

ISBN: 978-14051-4896-2

Library of Congress Cataloging-in-Publication Data

UCL Hospitals injectable medicines administration guide / Pharmacy
Department. – 2nd ed.
p. ; cm.
Includes bibliographical references.
ISBN-13: 978-1-4051-4896-2 (pbk. : alk. paper)
ISBN-10: 1-4051-4896-9 (pbk. : alk. paper)
1. Injections–Handbooks, manuals, etc. 2. Drugs–Handbooks, manuals,
etc. I. University College London Hospitals Foundation NHS Trust. Pharmacy
Dept. II. Title: Injectable medicines administration guide.
[DNLM: 1. Pharmaceutical Preparations–administration & dosage–Handbooks.
2. Injections, Intramuscular–methods–Handbooks. 3. Injections, Intravenous–
methods–Handbooks. 4. Injections, Subcutaneous–methods–Handbooks. QV 735
U17 2007]
RM170.U255 2007
615'.6–dc22
2006033544

A catalogue record for this title is available from the British Library

Set in Times Ten 10/12 pt
by SNP Best-set Typesetter Ltd., Hong Kong
Printed and bound in Singapore
by Markono Print Media Pte Ltd

The publisher's policy is to use permanent paper from mills that operate a sustainable
forestry policy, and which has been manufactured from pulp processed using acid-free
and elementary chlorine-free practices. Furthermore, the publisher ensures that the
text paper and cover board used have met acceptable environmental accreditation
standards.

For further information on Blackwell Publishing, visit our website:
www.blackwellnursing.com

CONTENTS

CONTRIBUTORS

Mr Gary Beacham

Mr Simon Cheesman, BPharm, MRPharmS

Mr Simon Clare, BA, RGN

Mr Geoff Cusack, FIPEM

Ms Julie Firth, BA, MSc, RGN, RHV

Mr Shahid Gani, BSc, MRPharmS

Ms Olivia Hameer, BSc, MRPharmS

Ms Jenni Hodgkinson, BSc

Mr Simon Keady, BSc, MRPharmS

Ms Fiona Maguire, BPharm, MRPharmS

Ms Anna Osadcow, MRPharmS

Ms Preet Panesar, BPharm, MRPharmS

Ms Sheetal Rambhai, BPharm, MRPharmS

Ms Liliana Singh, BSc, MRPharmS

ACKNOWLEDGEMENTS

The *UCL Hospitals Injectable Medicines Guide* is the result of an extensive team effort, some members of which have changed since the book was published within UCL Hospitals.

We would like to thank the listed contributors and to extend our thanks to other groups who provided helpful comments including the UCLH Use of Medicines Committee and the Nursing Practice Committee.

Furthermore, we acknowledge the UKCPA Critical Care Group for their Minimum Infusion Volume document (third edition). In addition we would like to acknowledge the contribution of Sarla Drayan, Robert Shulman, Simon Badcott, Mark Harries and Denise Hoare for their extensive work on the previous edition. We would also like to recognise the contribution of the Pharmacy Department of the Hammersmith Hospitals NHS Trust and to Susan Keeling and the pharmacists from many diferent hospitals from around the UK who have contributed to the national 'IV Guide' website. Information on the 'IV Guide' site can be obtained from Gill Bullock (gbullock@hhnt.org) who is based in the Pharmacy at Charing Cross Hospital.

The *UCL Hospitals Injectable Medicines Administration Guide Second Edition* is a fully revised and updated version of the previous edition published in 1997. Due to positive feedback obtained from pharmacists, nurses and doctors over the years, the general structure and format remain unchanged.

Over 20 new monographs have been included in this edition, ranging from intravenous paracetamol to drotrecogin alfa (activated) infusion. Additional information relating to drug–drug compatibility has also been included, and more detail has been published on the use of the aseptic non-touch technique method of preparing injectable medicines; in addition details about infusion devices have received an extensive update. Minimum infusion volumes have been inserted (where known) which should aid in the administration of intravenous medicines in the fluid-restricted patient. Moreover, new local practice recommendations have been included, which may differ from advice in the summary of product characteristics. Although the information contained in the medicine monographs is aimed at adult patients, information to support administration to children has been included for certain medicines.

Any comments, criticisms, suggestions for improvement or advice on changes will be gratefully received. This feedback is essential to ensure that the *UCL Hospitals Injectable Medicines Administration Guide* continues to be an accurate, useful, current, comprehensive and easy-to-use source of information.

Anthony Grosso
Formulary and Medicines Management Pharmacist
University College London Hospitals NHS Foundation Trust

Please send your comments to: anthony.grosso@uclh.nhs.uk

Section A

1. INTRODUCTION

The use of injectable medicines is part of everyday practice in hospitals and increasingly so in primary care. The relevant information needed for parenteral administration is often required in concise format in clinical areas. This need has prompted the publication of the *UCL Hospitals Injectable Medicines Administration Guide.*

The Guide includes information to support the prescribing, dispensing and administration of intravenous, subcutaneous and intramuscular medicines. It also includes a wealth of background information, including local policies and procedures, information relating to infusion devices and problems associated with injectable medicines.

2. EXPLANATORY NOTES OF INFORMATION IN THE MONOGRAPHS

2.1 ORGANISATION OF INFORMATION IN THE GUIDE

There are two sections in the *UCL Hospitals Injectable Medicines Administration Guide*.

Section A includes general information. This section includes explanatory notes on the abbreviations used and the type of information included, the responsibility of different professional groups, preparation on wards, guidance on flushing lines and cannulae, infusion pumps, discharge information, management of extravasation, syringe pump compatibility and pharmaceutical aspects of intravenous therapy.

Section B contains the individual medicine monographs in tabular form. Medicines are arranged in alphabetical order and the following information is included:

- Formulation
- Injectable method of administration
- Preparation of the medicine
- Administration details
- Stability
- Compatibility
- pH
- Suitable solutions for flushing as appropriate
- Sodium content
- Displacement value
- Acute bedside monitoring guidance
- Infusion device recommendation.

This Guide does not include information on cytotoxic medicines or those solely administered by the intramuscular or subcutaneous route.

2.2 SOURCES OF INFORMATION

The information and advice in the *UCL Hospitals Injectable Medicines Administration Guide* is based on the best available published data at the time of writing. Note, however, that published compatibility data are **not** available for all the combinations and situations covered in this guide. Some of the advice and information therefore reflects local practice and experience only. In addition, readers are reminded that slight variation in the exact combination and concentrations of medicines can adversely affect compatibility. Readers are referred to their local hospital pharmacy department for more specific information and advice. Neither the authors nor the publisher can accept any legal responsibility or liability for any errors or omissions that may be made. Readers should take their own precautions to ensure that new information published after the book was written is followed wherever possible. Readers are referred to the 'summary of product characteristics' (SPC or data sheets) produced by the pharmaceutical companies for further or more up-to-date information. SPCs are periodically updated and thus the recommendation(s) for administering the medicines included in this guide may alter from time to time.

2.3 USEFUL WEBSITES

Nurses
www.uclh.nhs.uk/News/2003/October/

www.nmc-uk.org

Pharmacists
www.ukcpa.org

All readers
www.bnf.org

www.bnfc.org

www.medicines.org

www.npsa.nhs.uk

www.mhra.gov.uk – useful documentation can be found by going to Publications/Safety Guidance/Device Bulletins

2.4 ABBREVIATIONS USED IN THIS GUIDE

2.4.1 Methods of administration

Abbreviation	Method of administration	Definition/description
(C) IV infusion	Continuous intravenous infusion	Intravenous administration of a volume of fluid with or without medicines added over a number of hours to achieve a given clinical endpoint. The infusion may be repeated over a period of days. Large-volume i.e. 250–1000 mL or small-volume infusions (e.g. 50 mL) may be delivered continuously
(I) IV infusion	Intermittent intravenous infusion	Administration of an infusion over a set time period, either as a one-off dose or repeated at specific time intervals
IV bolus	Intravenous bolus	Introduction of a small volume of medicine solution into the cannula or the injection site of an administration set. A bolus injection should be administered over 3–5 minutes unless otherwise specified
S/C	Subcutaneous injection	
(C) S/C infusion	Continuous subcutaneous infusion	
IM	Intramuscular injection	

2.4.2 Fluids

Abbreviation	Fluid
N/S	Sodium chloride 0.9% BP (normal or physiological saline)
G	Glucose 5% BP (dextrose 5%)
W	Water for injection (preservative free) BP
G/S	Glucose 4% and sodium chloride 0.18% BP
H	Compound sodium lactate (Hartmann's)
Ringer's	Ringer's solution
Hep/S	Heparin 10 units in 1 mL sodium chloride 0.9% – heparinised sodium chloride (e.g. Hepsal, Heplok)

2.5 'ACUTE EVENTS THAT MAY ACCOMPANY ADMINISTRATION'

Acute events that may accompany administration have been detailed where possible to warn the nurse or doctor administering the medicine of the most common adverse effects that may occur at the time (or immediately after) administration. The events listed are not comprehensive and do not cover delayed side effects or those that cannot be monitored at the bedside.

2.6 INTRAVENOUS MEDICINE COMPATIBILITY INFORMATION

As information is limited, medicines should ideally be infused separately.

The medicine compatibility section in the administration table contains information that is mainly based on physical compatibility, i.e. no visible sign of incompatibility after about four hours. When two medicines are described as Y-site compatible it is assumed that standard concentrations of both medicines are being mixed in a line and not in an infusion bag, burette or syringe. The compatibility information is not definitive, because varying the medicine concentration may produce signs of incompatibility (e.g. cloudiness, change in colour, haze or precipitation). This section has been left blank where there is no useful compatibility information available at the time of going to print. The medicines included in the compatibility section are not comprehensive and refer only to likely combinations of medicines used at UCL Hospitals.

Where two medicines are infused simultaneously via a Y site, the distal portion of the line should be examined for signs of incompatibility.

When using the compatibility information, ensure that both medicines are compatible with the infusion fluids in use.

Readers are referred to their local hospital pharmacy department with regard to medicine compatibility combinations that are not addressed in this Guide and for further information on a given combination.

2.7 pH VALUES

2.7.1 Incompatibility

The pH values are included to help predict possible physical incompatibility among medicines where no compatibility information exists. It is not advisable to administer medicines with widely differing pH values simultaneously because this may result in incompatibility, leading to precipitation or inactivation of either or both medicines.

2.7.2 Irritancy

The pH values are also used to indicate the irritancy of a medicine; see Section 7.2.3 (page 16) for full details.

2.8 DISPLACEMENT VALUES

Where the dose of a medicine is less than a complete vial and the vial requires reconstitution, e.g. for paediatrics, it is necessary to take into account the displacement value of the medicine.

For example:
To give a dose of 125 mg amoxicillin from a 250 mg vial:
The displacement value of amoxicillin 250 mg is 0.2 mL.
If 4.8 mL of diluent is added to a 250 mg vial, the volume of the resulting solution is 5 mL (i.e. 4.8 mL + 0.2 mL).
Therefore 125 mg will be contained in 2.5 mL of the solution.

3.1 RESPONSIBILITIES OF PROFESSIONAL STAFF AT UCLH

3.1.1 Nurses' responsibilities for injectable medicines (including blood products, IV fluids and IV medicines)

Nurses are referred to the *Guidelines for the Administration of Medicines* of the Nursing and Midwifery Council.

At UCL Hospitals, injectable medicines may be prepared and administered by a registered nurse/midwife as described in UCL Hospitals' *Administration of Medicines by Nurses/Midwives Policy and Procedure* document. This document is available from UCL Hospitals.

3.1.2 Pharmacists' responsibilities for injectable medicines

❏ Pharmacists monitor prescriptions for parenteral medicines and alert medical and/or nursing staff to any potential problems. Pharmacists should annotate prescriptions for parenteral medicines where appropriate.
❏ Pharmacists should provide appropriate information and advice to medical, nursing and other health professionals on all the pharmaceutical aspects of parenteral medicines, e.g. choice of medical therapy, compatibility, stability, dosage and administration details.
❏ Pharmacists provide education and training to healthcare professionals involved in the administration of parenteral medicines.
❏ A pharmacy will prepare complex medicines to be administered by the parenteral route as locally agreed.

3.2 PREPARATION OF INJECTABLE MEDICINES ON WARDS, CLINICS AND DEPARTMENTS AT UCLH

Injectable medicines:
❏ **must not** be prepared in advance of their immediate use
❏ **must not** be prepared by anyone other than the registered nurse/midwife or doctor who is going to administer them, unless they are prepared in his or her presence.

All medicines prepared must be appropriately labelled. Additive labels should be completed and attached to the infusion container.

Exceptions:

Injectable medicines may be prepared in advance only if covered by a specific protocol agreed by relevant pharmacy and nursing staff.

3.3 CHECKLIST FOR PREPARATION AND ADMINISTRATION OF INTRAVENOUS MEDICINES

❏ Pre-plan before drawing up doses
❏ Be sure of local protocols
❏ Check medicine against the prescription – check that the dose, time and route are correct
❏ Check patient identification
❏ Check IV site
❏ Check that any equipment required is working
❏ Know how to administer each medicine, e.g.
  – calculation of concentration and rate
  – reconstitution
  – addition of medicines to recommended diluents
  – check package insert, SPC, Pharmacy Medicines Information Centre or ward-based clinical pharmacist for further information
❏ Use aseptic technique during reconstitution steps, addition of medicine to diluents and care of the line (see 'ANTT' below)
❏ Maintain a sterile, particle-free solution
❏ Thoroughly mix any additions, checking for precipitation or particles
❏ Complete yellow infusion additive label and attach to infusion
❏ Understand how the medicine works and explain this to the patient if appropriate
❏ Continue to monitor for precipitation, patient response or adverse effects where appropriate.

3.4 ASEPTIC NON-TOUCH TECHNIQUE (ANTT)

The ANTT is a proven evidence-based method for standardising the aseptic technique of healthcare workers.

It is a simple, efficient and logical approach to IV therapy which is the same for peripheral and central line access and for all patients. In IV therapy the focus is on achieving asepsis of the 'key parts' at all the preparation and administration stages.

Key parts are those parts of the equipment that come into direct or indirect contact with the liquid infusion.

Healthcare workers should identify all key parts and then protect them at all times using a non-touch technique. On top of this fundamental principle, the ANTT guideline, importantly, standardises all the equipment to be used, and the order in which the procedure is performed. Standardisation is paramount.

ANTT guidelines and resources can be found at www.uclh.nhs/News/2003/October/. At UCLH, the ANTT picture guideline is displayed in all IV clinical areas. Here is a simple written overview of the ANTT guideline for IV therapy:

1. Gather equipment, medication, diluents, etc.
2. Clean aseptic field (plastic tray) with an alco-surface cleaner
3. Clean hands with alco-gel or soap and water
4. Put on non-sterile gloves
5. Prepare medicines and equipment, protecting key parts at all times by a non-touch technique
6. Go straight to the patient without interruption
7. Prepare the patient and gain free access to the IV line
8. If gloves are contaminated by this point, remove them, clean hands and put on new non-sterile gloves
9. Administer medicines – protecting key parts at all times
10. Dispose of equipment
11. Remove gloves
12. Wash hands.

4.1 FLUSHING BETWEEN MEDICINES

Flushing between administration of individual medicines must be carried out to avoid interaction between incompatible medicines. Unless the medicines concerned are known to be compatible, flushing between them must be undertaken.

Cannulae: 5–10 mL of either sodium chloride 0.9% (N/S) or glucose 5% (G) can be used for flushing. Check the individual medicine monograph for details of which flushing solution to use. Neonates usually require between 0.5 and 1 mL.

Lines: after medicine administration via an infusion line, the line should be flushed by connecting a bag containing one of the compatible infusion fluids. This should be administered at a rate not exceeding that recommended for administration of the original medicine. Approximately 20 mL must be infused, preferably from a 500 mL bag of sodium chloride 0.9% or glucose 5%, which is cheaper than a 100 mL bag. Neonates usually require between 1.0 and 2 mL.

4.2 FLUSHING CANNULAE NOT IN USE

Peripheral cannulae: flush 5 mL sodium chloride 0.9% 8 hourly to maintain patency of peripheral cannulae where there is no continuous infusion, unless medicines are being administered through the cannula at 8-hourly intervals or more frequently. Neonates usually require between 0.5 and 1 mL.

Central lines: UCL Hospitals staff follow a locally produced, skin-tunnelled, central line catheter policy.

Fatal errors have been reported after the incorrect administration of medicines via infusion pumps. It is the responsibility of the person administering the medicine to ensure that an appropriate pump is being used, that it is in good working order and that he or she knows how to operate it correctly. Alterations to the pump settings must be made by a person authorised to administer intravenous medicines. The volume of fluid administered should be recorded on the fluid chart. All pumps should be checked at least hourly during the infusion.

5.1 CHOICE OF PUMPS USED AT UCLH

In addition to the generic pumps described below, there are a number of special purpose pumps in use in specific clinical areas (e.g. the Cane ApoGo pump used for the administration of apomorphine in Parkinson's disease). These specialised pumps must be used **only** for their intended application; they must **not** be used as general purpose devices.

5.1.1 Volumetric pumps *(Alaris 591, 597, 598; Graseby 500)*

These are the preferred pumps for medium- and large-volume infusions, although some are designed specifically to operate at low flow rates for neonatal use. The rate is selected in millilitres per hour (usual range 1–999 mL/hour). Typically, most volumetric pumps are accurate to ±5% at rates down to 5 mL/hour. A syringe pump should be used for rates lower than 5 mL/hour. Volumetric pumps require the use of an administration set matched to the pump.

5.1.2 Syringe pumps *(e.g. Graseby 3100, 3300, 3400; Alaris P1000, P2000, Asena GH and CC)*

These are low-volume, high-accuracy devices designed to infuse at low flow rates and are typically calibrated for delivery in millilitres per hour (usual range 0.1–99 mL/hour). Many pumps will accept different sizes and different brands of syringe, but the pumps must be set up for the particular type and size of syringe in use, unless the pump detects the syringe size and type automatically. The Medicines and Healthcare Products Regulatory Agency (MHRA) recommends that rates

11

<0.5 mL/hour should not be used unless the pump is specially designed for this purpose, because an increase in the occlusion response time occurs. Where the response time to occlusion or the size of the post-occlusion bolus is important (e.g. in neonatal applications), syringe pumps allowing finer control over occlusion pressure should be used. These will generally require the use of a dedicated administration set (extension line) incorporating a pressure cell.

5.1.3 Pumps for ambulatory use

i. Miniature syringe pumps (syringe drivers) *(Graseby MS16 blue, MS26 green)*

These pumps typically accept syringes between 2 and 10 mL and are able to achieve very low flow rates of delivery. They may require the rate to be set in **millimetres** per **hour** or **millimetres** per **day**, i.e. linear travel of syringe plunger against time. Calculations that depend on the syringe size used are required to convert from flow rate to linear travel per unit time.

ii. Miniature volumetric pumps *(Graseby 9100, 9300, Walkmed 350)*

These pumps use reservoirs that contain the solution within the pump. Some offer a variety of programming options.

5.1.4 Patient-controlled analgesia (PCA) pumps
(Graseby 3300 PCA)

They are typically syringe pumps, but they have the facility to enable patients to administer a bolus dose to themselves. A PCA pump has several programming options, which may be set by specified clinical staff; access to the programming controls is usually restricted, typically by a key that disables the programming buttons. The syringe is generally contained inside a lockable cover, to prevent unauthorised access. With PCA pumps, protection against free flow is important, because the patient may be unsupervised for some of the time.

A different type of PCA device involves the use of an elastomeric reservoir (Baxter PCA) or syringe reservoir (Vygon PCA). Unlike electronic PCA pumps they have no programming features.

5.1.5 Target-controlled anaesthesia (TCI or TIVA) pumps
(Graseby 3500)

These are syringe pumps incorporating specialised software to control the delivery of specific anaesthetic agents, such as propofol (Diprivan). The pumps share most properties with syringe pumps but, instead of specifying a fixed infusion rate and volume directly, the user either sets an induction rate and volume, and a maintenance rate, or enters patient information such as gender and weight, from which the pump computes the required rates. The calculation is based on a pharmacokinetic model of the medicine's behaviour in the patient, and is intended to deliver the correct concentration in the patient. Note that some TCI/TIVA pumps require the medicine to be contained in a special, pre-filled syringe.

6. DISCHARGE INFORMATION FOR COMMUNITY NURSES INVOLVED IN THE ADMINISTRATION OF IV MEDICINES

Increasingly, patients are discharged on IV therapy for use at home. Often the task of IV administration falls to community nurses. Although community nurses may have access to their own IV administration policies and training, they often work in isolation and may not be familiar with the IV medicines that they are asked to administer.

Community nurses may therefore require information and advice on the IV medicine(s) before visiting the patient at home. Some may wish to visit the patient on the ward before discharge to familiarise themselves with the medicine, the type of equipment and/or the skills required for care. The information required by the community nurse will include:

❏ Name of medication
❏ Indication for use
❏ Dose
❏ Patient weight/body surface area/clinical status (as appropriate)
❏ Method of administration
❏ For IV infusions – diluent and volume/concentrations/rate/duration of infusion
❏ Method of rate control
❏ Frequency of administration (community nurse schedules and patient convenience may need consideration)
❏ Storage requirements
❏ Arrangements for ongoing prescription and supply of medicines
❏ Arrangements for disposal of clinical waste
❏ Side effects
❏ Clinically significant interactions
❏ Monitoring
❏ Reconstitution in the patient's home may pose additional training needs and COSHH (control of substances hazardous to health) implications must be considered.

For licensed products the above information will usually be available from the BNF, SPCs and package inserts. Where medicines are prescribed outside the recommendations of the product licence, community nurses require access to sufficient information to satisfy themselves that the prescription is appropriate in the context of the condition of the patient. The necessary information should be made available at the time of discharge from the ward. Prescribing guidelines, shared care guidelines and pharmacy discharge plans are a useful source of information.

7. MANAGEMENT OF EXTRAVASATION OF IV MEDICINES

Extravasation is the accidental infiltration of intravenous fluids into the subcutaneous tissue. It can occur for a number of reasons and may lead to an inflammatory response and/or pain from the affected tissue, which may be immediate or delayed. *The potential for a delayed reaction should be remembered when the initial assessment of a suspected extravasation site is made.*

It has been shown in several studies that a patient's risk of extravasation depends on several factors.

7.1 PATIENT FACTORS AFFECTING EXTRAVASATION

Certain groups of patients are more likely to develop problems after extravasation, and should therefore be monitored closely, including the following.

7.1.1 Neonates

Neonates, particularly pre-term neonates, possess less subcutaneous tissue than adults, and their veins are smaller and in some cases more fragile. In addition, any extravasated material is more concentrated in the affected area. They are also much less able to vocalise their pain (see below).

7.1.2 Patients unable to vocalise/communicate their pain

Comatose, anaesthetised patients and those being resuscitated are not able to provide clear vocalisation of the pain caused by the extravasation of a substance. They (and the neonates mentioned above) form perhaps the group of patients at greatest risk from extravasation.

7.1.3 Patients unable to sense pain

Special care should also be taken when administering IV medicines to patients who have an impaired ability to detect pain. Patients who suffer from peripheral neuropathy (e.g. people with diabetes) are one such group.

15

7.2 MEDICINE FACTORS AFFECTING EXTRAVASATION

7.2.1 Cytotoxic medicines

Several cytotoxic agents will cause extensive tissue damage if extravasated. Some of these agents require specific treatment when extravasation occurs (such advice is outside the scope of this guide).

7.2.2 Vasoconstrictor medicines

When these medicines are administered peripherally, extravasation can produce local vasoconstriction, leading to severe tissue hypoxia and ischaemia.

7.2.3 Irritant medicines

The following factors need to be considered before giving an intravenous medicine.

i. pH

Solutions with a high or low pH have the potential to cause more tissue damage if they are extravasated. The table on page 17 shows examples of medicines that have notably high or low pHs.

ii. Osmolarity

Solutions with an osmolarity greater than that of plasma (>290 mosmol/L) may cause tissue damage. The presence of these solutions can lead to an osmotic imbalance across the cell membrane, a breakdown of cellular transport mechanisms and cell death. Most IV medicines are formulated to have equal osmotic pressure as plasma, so that the solution to be injected into the patient is unlikely to cause disturbance to the tissues. The table on page 17 lists a selection of the medicines included in the *UCL Hospitals Injectable Medicines Administration Guide* that have high osmolarity and may potentially cause a problem if extravasated. Extra care should be taken when administering these medicines.

MEDICINES WITH HIGH OR LOW pH VALUES

Intravenous medicine	pH	Intravenous medicine	pH
Acetazolamide	9.2	Labetalol	3.5–4.2
Aciclovir	11	Lidocaine	3.5–6
Adrenaline (epinephrine)	2.5–3.6	Liothyronine	9.8–11.2
Allopurinol	10.8–11.8	Methoxamine	4.4
Aminophylline	8.8–10	Methyldopa	3–4.2
Amiodarone	3.5–4.5	Metoclopramide	3–7
Argipressin	2.5–5.4	Midazolam	3
Atracurium	3.5	Morphine	3–6
Atropine	3–4.5	Naloxone	3–4.5
Azathioprine	10–12	Noradrenaline (norepinephrine) acid tartrate	3–4.5
Buprenorphine	3.5–5.5	Octreotide	3.9–4.5
Cholecystokinin (CCK)	3–6	Omeprazole	9–10
Clonazepam	3.5–4.5	Ondansetron	3.3–4
Co-trimoxazole	9–10.5	Oxytocin	3.7–4.3
Cyclizine	3.3–3.7	Pancuronium	3.8–4.2
Dantrolene	9.5	Papaveretum	2.5–4
Diazoxide	11.6	Phenobarbital (phenobarbitone)	9–10.5
Dobutamine	2.5–5.5	Phenoxybenzamine	2.5–3.1
Dopamine	2.5–5.5	Phenytoin sodium	12
Doxapram	3–5	Potassium canrenoate	10.7–11.2
Droperidol	2.7–4.7	Prochlorperazine	5.5–6.6
Ergometrine	2.7–3.5	Propranolol	3
Fentanyl	4–7.5	Protamine sulphate	2.5–3.5
Folic acid	8–11	Quinine dihydrochloride	1.5–3
Furosemide	8–9.5	Salbutamol	3.5
Ganciclovir	10–11	Secretin	2.5–5
Gentamicin	3–5	Sodium nitroprusside	3.5–6
Glucagon	2.5–3.5	Sulfadiazine	11
Glucose (pH dependent on concentration of solution)	3.5–6.5	Terbutaline	3–5
Glyceryl trinitrate	3.5–6.5	Tetracosactide	3.8–4.5
Glycopyrronium	2.3–4.3	Tetracycline	1.8
Haloperidol	3–3.8	Thiamine	2.5–4.5
Hydralazine	3.5–4.2	Thiopental	10.5
Hyoscine butylbromide	3.7–5.5	Tobramycin	3.5–6
Ketamine	3.5–5.5	Vancomycin	2.8–4.5

This is not a comprehensive list.

MEDICINES WITH HIGH OSMOLARITY

Intravenous medicine	Osmolarity (mosmol/L)	Intravenous medicine	Osmolarity (mosmol/L)
Glucose 10%	535	Mannitol 10%	550
Glucose 20%	1110	Mannitol 20%	1100
Glucose 50%	2775	Magnesium sulphate 50%	4060
Calcium gluconate 10%	670	Potassium chloride 20mmol/10mL	4000
Calcium chloride 5mmol/10mL	1500	Sodium bicarbonate 4.2%	1004
TPN/IVN bags	>290 (variable with bag contents)	Sodium bicarbonate 8.4%	2008

This is not a comprehensive list.

7.2.4 Vasoactive medicines

As a result of their direct vasoconstrictive action on blood vessels, medicines such as adrenaline (epinephrine), noradrenaline (norepinephrine), dobutamine, dopamine and vasopressin will reduce the ability of blood vessels in the extravasated area to allow blood to flow freely. This may result in ischaemic injury to the area concerned. If the ischaemia is prolonged or severe, necrosis may develop in the extravasated area.

7.3 ADMINISTRATION FACTORS AFFECTING EXTRAVASATION

7.3.1 Site of administration

The selection of the site is a very important factor when administering an IV medicine. Areas that have small amounts of subcutaneous tissue are the most likely to be problematic should the medicine extravasate. The antecubital fossa and the dorsum of the hand and foot are most often implicated in extravasation injury and should be avoided when administering irritant or vasoactive medicines and those capable of causing discharge or blistering.

7.3.2 Method of venepuncture

This is probably as important as the site of injection. The repeated use of any single vein for venepuncture increases the risk of the medicine extravasating to the surrounding tissues. *Venepuncture is a skill that should not be attempted by anybody who has not completed an approved training course.* Inexperience increases the risk of problems arising from venepuncture.

7.4 TREATMENT OF EXTRAVASATION

Extravasation should be suspected if:

❏ Patient complains of burning, stinging or any discomfort at the injection site
❏ Swelling or leakage is observed at the injection site
❏ Resistance is felt on the plunger of the syringe (if the medicine is being given as a bolus)

❏ There is an absence of free flow of fluid if an infusion is in progress.

7.4.1 Immediate action

❏ **STOP** the administration of the medicine, **leaving the cannula in place**.
❏ Aspirate the residual medicine through the cannula.
❏ Elevate the limb.
❏ Inform the medical staff immediately.

At UCL Hospitals the medical/surgical team refer all cases to the plastic surgery team for assessment and advice on treatment at the *earliest opportunity*. The plastic surgery team have several techniques available to them to limit the likelihood of extensive tissue damage after extravasation. The sooner these measures are started, the more successful they are likely to be.

7.4.2 Subsequent action

Careful recording of the following in the medical (and nursing) notes is recommended:

❏ Medicine(s) involved
❏ Appearance of site
❏ Date and time of the incident
❏ Administration technique
❏ Needle size, type and insertion site
❏ Patient's symptoms and statements
❏ Approximate amount of medicine extravasated
❏ Name and signature of nurse/doctor administering the medicine
❏ Doctor notified
❏ Time and date of referral to plastic surgery team
❏ Follow-up procedure.

The doctor/nurse administering the medicine should complete an adverse incident form as per trust policy and any other documentation necessary for patient problems.

Continuous subcutaneous infusions are commonly used in palliative care. It is sometimes necessary to give more than one medicine by this method. However, not all medicines are suitable for subcutaneous administration because of limited aqueous solubility or extremes of pH. The following simple precautions will minimise the risk of problems of incompatibility and instability:

- Do not leave any medicines running in a syringe pump for more than 24 hours
- Protect contents of syringe from direct sunlight
- Ensure that solution appears clear and colourless with no signs of precipitation or crystallisation
- Check with your local pharmacy department for specific stability information before using any unusual combinations
- The pH is a useful predictor of compatibility of medicine combinations. If two medicines with differing pH values are mixed, the solubility and chemical stability of combinations may be affected.

Please refer to the current trust (*or* your local) syringe driver policy for further information on the use of syringe drivers.

The table opposite shows the maximum stable concentrations of **diamorphine** (a commonly used opioid in the palliative care setting) with various agents, made up with **water for injection** (unless otherwise stated). At concentrations above those shown, there is an increased potential for the mixture to precipitate.

Additive	Maximum stable concentration of additive in syringe pump (mg/mL)	Maximum stable concentration of diamorphine in syringe pump (mg/mL)	See note
Cyclizine	10	50	1
Dexamethasone sodium phosphate	1.6	50	2
Haloperidol	1.5	50	
Hyoscine butylbromide	20	150	
Hyoscine hydrobromide	0.4	150	
Ketamine			3
Levomepromazine (methotrimeprazine)	10	50	4
Metoclopramide	5	150	5
Midazolam	5	43	
Ketorolac	12	400	6
Octreotide	0.075	25	3

Notes

1 Cyclizine is likely to precipitate in the presence of sodium chloride 0.9%. In addition, the solubility of cyclizine is reduced by the presence of other medicines in solution. Check for precipitation before administration. Certain higher concentrations of cyclizine may be compatible with lower concentrations of diamorphine. Contact pharmacy for details.
2 Check for precipitation before administration. Dexamethasone should be added last to the syringe after dilution of other medicines.
3 The maximum compatible concentrations of this combination are not known. No formal stability studies have been published. Sodium chloride 0.9% is the preferred diluent for these combinations.
4 Solutions containing levomepromazine have developed a purple discoloration in UV light: such solutions should be discarded.
5 Under some conditions metoclopramide may become discoloured: such solutions should be discarded.
6 Ketorolac and diamorphine should be mixed in sodium chloride 0.9%. The 'maximum' concentrations stated are the maximum concentrations reported in the literature. The absolute maximum compatible concentrations of ketorolac and diamorphine are not known.

9. CHOICE OF ROUTE OF ADMINISTRATION

9.1 BENEFITS OF INTRAVENOUS ROUTE

The intravenous route has a number of hazards associated with it, and must never be considered lightly. It should be used only if no other route of administration is appropriate. Situations in which intravenous therapy would be appropriate are when:

❑ The patient is unable to take oral medication, absorb the medicine or tolerate the medication orally
❑ High medicine levels are required that cannot be achieved rapidly by another route
❑ Sustained medicine levels need to be maintained (such as those achieved by a continuous infusion)
❑ Some medicines cannot be given by another route because of their chemical properties (e.g. are not absorbed from the gut, inactivated by the gut or not released from muscle)
❑ An immediate response is required.

Medicines administered intravenously avoid having to undergo the process of absorption into the bloodstream compared with other routes, e.g. oral medicines are absorbed via the gut mucosa and medicines administered intramuscularly have to be absorbed from the muscle fibres into the bloodstream.

9.2 IMPACT OF THE FIRST-PASS EFFECT

Medicines given orally are usually absorbed in the small intestine and enter the portal system to the liver where they may be metabolised. For some medicines, metabolism in the liver occurs to such a great extent that little medicine reaches the target organ – this is called the first-pass effect (or first-pass metabolism). Therefore the oral dose for a similar therapeutic effect may need to be higher, e.g. verapamil, propranolol, glyceryl trinitrate. For some medicines, e.g. lidocaine, it is not possible to make an oral formulation because the metabolism is so great.

9.3 IMPACT OF HALF-LIFE

The elimination half-life $(t_{1/2})$ is the time taken for the concentration of medicine in the blood or plasma to fall to half its original value, e.g. if a medicine has a half-life of 4 hours, this means that it will take 4 hours for the concentration of the medicine in the blood to fall from, for example, 10 mg/L to 5 mg/L. Medicines can have half-lives that are measured in seconds, minutes, hours or days.

Medicines with very short half-lives disappear from the bloodstream very quickly and may need to be administered by a continuous infusion to maintain a clinical effect on tissues, e.g. dopamine has a half-life of 1–2 minutes and so has to be given as a continuous infusion. When the infusion is stopped its effects will be lost within minutes.

If a medicine has a longer half-life, it means that it may be able to be given as a bolus injection or intermittent infusion instead of a continuous infusion, and its effects on the body tissues will last for several hours before another dose is needed. Knowledge of half-life alone is not, however, sufficient in determining the method of administration because many other factors need to be taken into consideration, e.g. drug distribution.

9.4 ADVANTAGES AND DISADVANTAGES OF INTRAVENOUS ADMINISTRATION

Advantages
❏ Rapid response achievable (e.g. cardiac arrest)
❏ Constant therapeutic effect achievable (e.g. continuous infusion)
❏ To allow medicine administration when the oral route cannot be used (e.g. nil-by-mouth [NBM] patients at risk of aspiration or nausea and vomiting)
❏ IM route inappropriate (e.g. small muscle mass, thrombocytopenic, haemophiliacs)
❏ To achieve effects unattainable by oral administration (e.g. medicine metabolised extensively, non-absorption of medicine)
❏ To enable medicines to be administered to patients who are unconscious
❏ To allow fluid and electrolyte imbalance to be promptly corrected.

Disadvantages
❏ Increased risk of toxicity (side effects usually more immediate and severe)
❏ Risk of embolism

- Increased risk of microbial contamination/infection
- Risk of extravasation/phlebitis
- Risk of particulate contamination
- Administration hazards (e.g. pain on injection)
- Risk of fluid overload
- Problems with compatibility/stability of medicines

9.5 ROUTES OF INTRAVENOUS ADMINISTRATION

9.5.1 Peripheral versus central vein administration

Peripheral vein administration

Advantages
- Simple
- Cheap
- Less traumatic compared with central line
- Cannula easier to manage for clinical staff

Disadvantages
- Limited time period of use
- Blocks more easily
- Risk of infection
- Extravasation/phlebitis
- Single lumen
- Not suitable for certain medicines

Central vein administration

Advantages
- Administration of hypertonic fluids
- Administration of other irritant solutions, e.g. cytotoxics, total parental nutrition (TPN) or intravenous nutrition (IVN) inotopes, inotropes
- Rapid administration of large volumes, e.g. in shock
- Long-term venous access, e.g. cytotoxics, TPN/IVN
- To enable more concentrated solutions of medicines, which would normally need further dilution as a result of their irritancy, to be given in fluid/sodium-restricted patients, e.g. potassium chloride
- Administration of medicines with a pharmacological action on veins (such as vasoconstriction, e.g. dopamine)
- Cannulae can have more than one lumen (e.g. triple lumen), which prevents medicines mixing together

Disadvantages
❏ Morbidity associated with central line insertion
❏ Cannulae take time and skill to insert
❏ Skilled staff required to care for line
❏ High infection risk
❏ Expensive to insert

Medicines that must be administered centrally include adrenaline (epinephrine), noradrenaline (norepinephrine), dopamine and amiodarone.

10. METHODS OF INTRAVENOUS ADMINISTRATION

10.1 INTRAVENOUS BOLUS

Introduction of a small volume of medicine solution into a cannula or the injection site of an administration set is referred to as a bolus injection. A bolus injection should be administered over 3–5 minutes unless otherwise specified, e.g. adenosine, which is very rapidly inactivated and needs to be administered as quickly as possible.

Indications

❏ To achieve immediate and high medicine levels. This may be appropriate when time is limited or in cases of emergency.
❏ To ensure that medicines that are inactivated very rapidly, e.g. adenosine, produce a clinical effect.

Drawbacks

❏ Tendency to administer the dose too rapidly with potential for increased adverse effects.
❏ Damage to the veins, e.g. phlebitis or extravasation, especially with potentially irritant medicines.
❏ Volume of diluent recommended may not be practical for the time of administration.
❏ Injection is unlikely to be able to be stopped if an adverse event occurs.
❏ High rate of administration may be associated with increased adverse events for some medicines, e.g. vancomycin.

10.2 INTERMITTENT INTRAVENOUS INFUSION

Administration of an infusion over a set time period, either as a one-off dose or repeated at specific time intervals, is referred to as an intermittent infusion. An intermittent infusion of medicine is often a compromise between a bolus injection and continuous infusion. It achieves high plasma concentrations rapidly to ensure clinical efficacy and yet reduces the risks of adverse reactions associated with rapid administration.

10.3 CONTINUOUS INTRAVENOUS INFUSION

Intravenous administration of a volume of fluid with or without medicines added, over a number of hours, to achieve a clinical endpoint is referred to as a continuous infusion. The infusion may be repeated over a period of days. Large volumes, i.e. 250–1000 mL, or small-volume infusions (e.g. 50 mL) may be delivered continuously.

Indications

❏ When a constant therapeutic medicine concentration is required or when the plasma concentration needs to be maintained within tight limits.
❏ When a medicine has a short elimination half-life and can have an effect only if given continuously.

Drawbacks

❏ Volume of diluent may cause fluid overload in susceptible patients
❏ Incompatibility problems with the diluent
❏ Incomplete mixing of solutions
❏ Calculation skills required for accurate determination of infusion concentration and rates. Knowledge of, and competence in, operating infusion devices required
❏ Increased risk of microbial and particulate contamination during preparation
❏ Risk of phlebitis and extravasation
❏ Need for regular monitoring during infusion.

11. FORMULATION AND PRESENTATION OF INTRAVENOUS MEDICINES

Parenteral medicines differ in the presentations that are available.

11.1 MEDICINES THAT REQUIRE RECONSTITUTION

These include medicines, e.g. amoxicillin, that are presented as a dry powder and therefore need to be reconstituted before use. Further dilution may be necessary. The advantage of this type of formulation is that it enables prolonged storage of products that are unstable in solution.

There are a number of disadvantages, including the following:

- ❏ Reconstitution, which is time-consuming, particularly if the preparation is difficult to dissolve
- ❏ All manipulations pose the risk of environmental and microbial contamination of the solution
- ❏ Care may be required if the medicine is susceptible to 'foaming', because incomplete doses may be withdrawn, e.g. teicoplanin
- ❏ If the product is presented as glass ampoules that require snapping, there is a danger of glass particles getting into the preparation, staff injuries and the risk of medicine droplets polluting the environment
- ❏ Where vials are presented with a rubber septum, care must be taken to avoid pressure differentials when trying to introduce the diluent or withdrawing the reconstituted medicine.

Equalising pressure in vial

Some vials are manufactured with a vacuum inside, and it is important that the effects of this are corrected during reconstitution. If the vial has a vacuum inside, it will be obvious when trying to add diluent because the diluent will be 'sucked' into the vial.

If no vacuum is present in the vial, air needs to be removed. The amount of air drawn back into the syringe should be equal to the volume of diluent added. Before withdrawing the reconstituted medicine from the vial, again pressure differences have to be accounted for. Air needs to be added to the vial equal to the amount of medicine to be withdrawn.

28

11.2 PREPARATIONS IN SOLUTION REQUIRING FURTHER DILUTION BEFORE USE

Examples of such preparations are ranitidine and amiodarone.

The advantage of these preparations are that:

❑ They are already in a liquid form, so reconstitution is unnecessary.

The disadvantages include the following:

❑ Need for further dilution before administration may be time-consuming
❑ Prone to vacuum/pressure problems (if vials)
❑ Can cause glass breakage problems (if ampoules)
❑ Poses the risk of microbial contamination.

11.3 PREPARATIONS AVAILABLE 'READY TO USE' WITHOUT FURTHER DILUTION

These preparations may come in bags or small-volume ampoules that can be administered without further dilution, but still require the solution to be drawn up into a syringe for administration, e.g. adenosine, gentamicin, metoclopramide. These are convenient to use but still have the disadvantages of:

❑ Hazards associated with microbial contamination
❑ Prone to vacuum/pressure problems (if vials)
❑ Can cause glass breakage problems (if ampoules).

11.4 PREPARATIONS 'READY TO USE'

These preparations include infusion bags and pre-filled syringes, e.g. 500 mL sodium chloride 0.9%, morphine sulphate 60 mg in 60 mL PCA syringes. They have the advantages of:

❑ Lower risk of environmental contamination
❑ Minimal microbial contamination
❑ Being easy to use
❑ Being time saving.

12. PROBLEMS ASSOCIATED WITH IV MEDICINE ADMINISTRATION

12.1 PAIN ON IV INJECTION

This may be a sign of not following recommended administration advice – check manufacturer's literature, with your local pharmacy medicine information department or this Guide. It is also important to check the IV site itself for any problems.

Pain on injection can occur for a number of reasons. Hypertonicity, i.e. medicines that have a higher osmolarity than plasma (osmolarity >290 mosmol/L), can cause fluids to pass out of blood cells, resulting in cell dyormation or lysis. Inappropriate rapid administration or insufficient dilution of irritant medicines can result in damage to blood vessels and pain. If recommendations are being followed and pain is still a problem, try reducing the rate and/or increasing the dilution.

Pain can be caused by a wide variety of factors including pH, tonicity and chemical irritancy. Common examples of medicines that cause pain on injection are:

Erythromycin   Potassium infusions
Sodium bicarbonate 8.4%   Dextrose solutions >10%
Tetracycline   Phenytoin
Vancomycin

12.2 PHLEBITIS AND EXTRAVASATION

12.2.1 Phlebitis

This is a red, corded, inflamed vein which permits poor flow of blood or injected medicne.

12.2.2 Extravasation (infiltration, tissuing)

This is the accidental infiltration of intravenous fluids/medicines into the subcutaneous tissue (other causes may be physical or chemical). It can occur for a number of reasons and may lead to an inflammatory response and/or pain from the affected tissue, which may be immediate or delayed.

However, it can occur as a result of administration of an irritant medicine. This causes vasoconstriction and possibly occlusion of the vein resulting in a high back pressure and extravasation of the administered solution. The solution may leak out of the vein at the point where it was punctured by the cannula.

The most common examples of medicines that can cause more tissue damage if extravasated are given below. They are more likely to cause damage if they are hypertonic, chemical irritants or have a pH outside 4–8 (i.e. strongly acidic or alkaline).

For further information on the management of extravasation of intravenous medicines refer to Section A7.

12.3 FACTORS AFFECTING PATENCY OF IV SITES

12.3.1 Factors increasing failure of IV sites

❏ Infection
❏ Irritation:
  – movement
  – cannula material (steel is more irritant than Teflon)
  – particles (terminal in-line filters help)
  – irritant medicines, e.g. doxorubicin, diazepam, erythromycin, potassium infusions
  – pH appears to be an important factor; extremes of pH, i.e. high or low pH values, are more likely to be irritant.

12.3.2 Factors decreasing failure of IV sites

❏ In-line filters
❏ Good practice/aseptic technique
❏ Neutral solutions
❏ A number of interventions have been proposed to prolong the patency of IV lines, although the supporting evidence base is variable, e.g. heparin, topical steroids (blocks inflammatory mechanism) and glyceryl trinitrate patches (vasodilatation)

12.4 PROBLEMS WITH RAPID ADMINISTRATION

❏ Usually avoided if administration advice followed.
❏ Wide variety of problems could arise, e.g. fluid overload, excessive pharmacological action. Some common problems are listed overleaf.

Medicine	Problem
Furosemide	Increased risk of ototoxicity (deafness) at >4 mg/minute
Fusidic acid	Increased risk of haemolysis and hepatotoxicity
Vancomycin	Increased risk of red man syndrome[a] especially if given over <1 hour
Sulphonamides	Increased risk of crystalluria (crystals in the urine)
Cimetidine,[b] ranitidine	Arrhythmias, arrest
Theophylline	Arrhythmias, nausea, vomiting, tachycardia
Potassium chloride	Arrhythmias, cardiac arrest >20 mmol/hour
Lidocaine	Arrhythmias, arrest
Methylprednisolone sodium succinate	Cardiovascular collapse >50 mg/minute
Phenytoin	Arrhythmias, respiratory/cardiac arrest if administered at >50 mg/minute

[a]Red man syndrome is flushing (macular rash), fever, rigors.
[b]Cimetidine: arrhythmias appear to be more common compared with ranitidine.

12.5 FACTORS AFFECTING DROP SIZE

The presence of solvents in the medicine may affect the drop size of the infusion, e.g. amiodarone, etoposide. This can result in inaccuracies if relying on drop-counting methods to control the administration rate. Therefore, these medicines should be given only by devices controlled by volume (see Section 5).

12.6 HIGH SODIUM CONTENT

Some medicines can have a high sodium content that may need to be taken into consideration when patients are sodium restricted. Sodium may be in the medicine as the sodium salt or in the additives as a buffer, or may be used as the diluent, i.e. sodium chloride 0.9%.

Examples:

❏ Sodium salts and additives

	Na$^+$ content
Ceftazidime 2 g	4.6 mmol/vial
Ciprofloxacin	15.4 mmol/100 mL

❏ Diluent
  - IV metronidazole 500 mg = 13.2 mmol Na$^+$/100 mL bag
  - erythromycin depending on volume of sodium chloride 0.9% used as diluent (e.g. could be 2 L/day, i.e. 300 mmol Na$^+$)

12.7 FLUID RESTRICTION

Medicines that require dilution in large volumes for administration may cause problems in patients who are fluid restricted. Fluid overload may also arise where patients are being administered numerous intravenous medicines that may require dilution. Therefore, the amount of fluid intake from intravenous medicine administration must be considered when prescribing maintenance fluid requirements. In the monographs, advice has been inserted to indicate minimum volumes that can be used. Much of this information is based on anecdotal experience compiled in the UKCPA document *Critical Care Group Minimum Infusion Volume*, 3rd edn, 2006.

❏ High fluid intake often accompanies the following medicines:
  - co-trimoxazole (high dose)
  - sodium fusidate
  - cyclophosphamide
  - erythromycin
  - cisplatin
  - TPN/IVN regimens.

12.8 LAYERING

This phenomenon can occur if there is insufficient mixing of solutions with different densities. The best example of this is the addition of potassium chloride to IV infusion bags. If potassium chloride injection is added to glucose 5%, it remains in the bottom of the IV bag because it is denser than glucose. Thus, if the two solutions are not mixed thoroughly, there is a high concentration of potassium in the lower part of the IV bag – in this case cardiac arrest could occur as a high concentration of potassium would be delivered in a short space of time. Care must be taken to ensure that all additives are thoroughly mixed within the infusion fluid to which they have been added before administration.

13. FACTORS INFLUENCING MEDICINE STABILITY AND COMPATIBILITY OF IV MEDICINES

An important aspect of parenteral therapy is to ensure that the patient receives the intended dose of each medicine. A proportion of the medicine will be lost between the time of preparation of the injection and entry into the bloodstream, e.g. if the medicine undergoes degradation, precipitates with the diluent or interacts with the delivery system. It is important to understand the reasons for such losses of potency in order to assess the likely clinical implications.

The following section briefly discusses some of these problems.

13.1 DEGRADATION

13.1.1 In aqueous solution

Medicines, on reconstitution, are relatively unstable in aqueous vehicles and normally degrade by hydrolysis (decomposition of a substance by a chemical reaction with water). This reaction may be accelerated by a change in pH, resulting either from the diluent or from a second medicine. Such degradation may be minimised and prevented by using the recommended diluent, e.g. erythromycin must be reconstituted with water for injection because it will not dissolve in 0.9% sodium chloride or glucose and should then be diluted in 0.9% sodium chloride and not glucose because it degrades at an acidic pH.

13.1.2 Photodegradation

Photodegradation is the breakdown of a substance by light. It occurs to a significant degree in a small number medicines, e.g. vitamin A and sodium nitroprusside. Degradation is usually the result of UV light, which is found in daylight but not artificial fluorescent light. However, sodium nitroprusside is rapidly degraded by both fluorescent and UV light.

Photodegradation of some other light-sensitive medicines (e.g. ciprofloxacin or furosemide) is not clinically important provided that direct exposure to strong daylight or sunlight is avoided.

13.2 PRECIPITATION

Precipitated medicines are pharmacologically inactive but hazardous to the patient. Precipitates can block catheters and damage capillaries, and may lead to coronary and pulmonary emboli. The injection of medicine precipitates must therefore be avoided.

13.2.1 Causes of precipitation

pH

The most likely reason for precipitation is the mixing in the infusion container or the infusion line of two medicines with very different pH values, especially if one is acidic and the other alkaline.

Medicine–medicine co-precipitation

This occurs most commonly from the mixing of organic anions (ions with a negative charge) and cations (ions with a positive charge), which join together to form ion pairs. Examples include gentamicin and other aminoglycosides, heparin and some cephalosporins. It is essential to avoid these interactions. Medicines that could form an ion pair should never be allowed to mix in an infusion container, syringe or administration line, e.g. flush gentamicin with sodium chloride 0.9% before giving heparin.

Temperature

Most medicines are more soluble as the temperature increases. Generally, if a refrigerated injection does not precipitate, warming to 37°C (as occurs when an injection passes slowly through the cannula) will not cause precipitation. One exception to this is calcium phosphate, which is less soluble at 37°C than at room temperature.

Mannitol, at concentrations of 15% or more, crystallises out when exposed to low temperatures. A mannitol solution containing crystals should not be used.

13.3 BINDING OF MEDICINES TO PLASTICS

Administration of IV medicines relies almost entirely on equipment made from plastic. Some medicines bind to certain plastics. The extent of binding is difficult to predict because it depends on: medicine concentration, vehicle, flow rate, available surface area of plastic, type of plastic, temperature, pH and time.

The table below shows some clinically relevant examples.

Medicine	Plastic affected	Avoided by
Insulin	Any (and glass)	Not adding to infusion bags, give in syringe pump, at >1 unit/ml. Also monitor clinically
Diazepam	PVC	Not using PVC bags and sets. Use polyethylene extension sets and syringe pump (minor losses to syringes – change every 12–24 hours)
Nimodipine	PVC	Using polyethylene extension sets and syringe pump
Nitrates (GTN, ISDN)	PVC, nylon	Not using PVC bags and sets. Use polyethylene extension lines with syringe pumps or polyfusors
Clomethiazole	PVC, nylon	Not using PVC bags and sets. If PVC sets are used they must be changed at least every 24 hours

13.4 DESTABILISATION OF PARENTERAL EMULSIONS

Care is necessary to avoid destabilising emulsions in IV lines, junctions and catheters where many injections may mix during administration. Fat emulsions (e.g. Intralipid) are used widely in parenteral nutrition as an energy source. Other medicines that are prepared as a fat emulsion as a result of their poor water solubility include propofol and diazepam (Diazemuls).

Fat emulsions can be destabilised by ions with a high positive charge (e.g. calcium, magnesium) or by mixing calcium and heparin in the same IV line, e.g. in neonatal TPN/IVN. Diazemuls may be diluted, but sodium chloride 0.9% rapidly destabilises the emulsion and should not be used.

13.5 LEACHING OF PLASTICISERS

The presence of oils and surfactants can leach (leak) out toxic plasticisers, especially from PVC materials. This can happen if TPN/IVN is made in PVC bags. Leaching from administration sets and bags during infusion can also occur, e.g. for ciclosporin, the infusion should be used within 6 hours because the solution contains polyethoxylated castor oil, which causes phthalate (a plasticiser) to leach from PVC containers and tubing. If the infusion is administered for more than 6 hours, a low sorbing giving set and a glass bottle should be used to infuse the ciclosporin. Leaching from rubber plungers of plastic syringes may occur and can affect medicine stability, e.g. asparaginase.

13.6 BLOOD AND BLOOD PRODUCTS

The Department of Health states that the co-administration of blood or concentrated red blood cells with any other medicine or vehicle is hazardous. Examples of incompatibility with blood include mannitol solutions (irreversible crenation of red cells), dextrans (rouleaux formation and interference with crossmatching), glucose (clumping of red cells) and oxytocin (inactivated).

In extreme circumstances medicines have been mixed with blood in the catheter, e.g. experience seems to show that furosemide can mix safely with blood. In contrast, human serum albumin has been shown to be incompatible with many intravenous infusions. Overall experience remains limited and no studies have been reported.

13.7 ANAPHYLAXIS

A true allergic reaction resulting in anaphylaxis will occur in a patient who has become sensitised to a medicine, via an immunologically mediated pathway, and so must have had previous exposure to the medicine. Therefore, anaphylaxis will occur on administration of the second rather than the first dose of the medicine. In a patient already sensitised to a specific medication, the risk of an allergic reaction to that medication is greatest when given intravenously and least when given orally. This is thought to be a function of the rate of medicine delivery.

Pseudoallergic reactions are medicine reactions that exhibit clinical signs and symptoms of an allergic response, but are not immunologically mediated. Unlike true allergic reactions, which require an induction period during which a patient becomes sensitised to an antigen, pseudoallergic reactions can occur on the first exposure to a medicine. The development of pseudoallergic reactions may be dose related and manifest only when large doses of the medicine are administered.

Section B

Medicine monographs (in alphabetical order)

Abbreviations (See Section A, 2.4 for further details)

(C) IV infusion	Continuous intravenous infusion
(I) IV infusion	Intermittent intravenous infusion
IV bolus	Intravenous bolus
S/C	Subcutaneous injection
(C) S/C infusion	Continuous subcutaneous infusion
IM	Intramuscular injection
N/S	Sodium chloride 0.9% BP (normal or physiological saline)
G	Glucose 5% BP
W	Water for injection (preservative free) BP
G/S	Glucose 4% and sodium chloride 0.18% BP
H	Compound sodium lactate (Hartmann's)
Hep/S	Heparin 10 units in 1 mL sodium chloride 0.9% – heparinised sodium chloride (e.g. Hepsal)

Other abbreviations

APTT	Activated partial thromboplastin time
BM	Bone marrow
CAPD	Continuous ambulatory peritoneal dialysis
ICU	Intensive care unit
ITU	Intensive therapy unit
NBM	Nil by mouth
PBSC	Peripheral blood stem cells
PVC	Polyvinyl chloride
SPC	Summary of product characteristics

Formulation	Method	Dilution	Rate	Comments	Compatibility
Abciximab					
Vial 10 mg/5 mL	IV bolus (immediately followed by infusion)	Refer to specific product information for preparation and administration. Guidance given with the manufacturers' filter pack provided.	1 minute	**Acute events that may accompany administration:** Bleeding, particularly when cardiac catheterisation is via femoral access site; remove sheath when coagulation has returned to normal. Thrombocytopenia, especially on second exposure: monitor platelet count before and 2–4 hours after bolus dose, and in 24 hours if infusion is continued. Seek haematologist's advice if platelet count decreases. **pH:** 7.3 **Flush:** N/S or G **Displacement:** N/A **Sodium content:** Negligible **Other comments:** Use infusion within 24 hours.	Do not infuse with any other medicines.
	(C) IV infusion (immediately after bolus)	Refer to specific product information for preparation and administration. Guidance given with the manufacturers' filter pack provided.	Max. 10 micrograms/ minute		

Formulation	Method	Dilution	Rate	Comments	Compatibility
Acetazolamide					
Vial 500mg	IV bolus	Reconstitute each 500mg with at least 5mL W.	Usual maximum rate of between 100 and 500mg/minute	**Acute events that may accompany administration:** Extravasation may cause tissue damage; for management guidelines, see Section A, 7 **pH:** 9.2 **Flush:** N/S or G **Sodium content:** 2.36mmol/vial **Displacement:** 0.36mL/500mg. Add 4.64mL of diluent to 500mg vial to give a concentration of 500mg/5mL.	Do not infuse with other medicines.
	IM (not recommended as painful due to alkaline pH).	As above.			

- For abbreviations used in the Table, see Section A, 2.4.
  - e.g. (C) IV = continuous intravenous infusion; (I) IV = intermittent intravenous infusion.
  - Prepare a fresh infusion every 24hours unless otherwise specified.
  - Presume suitability as single-use only unless otherwise specified.
  - Always check with additional reference sources regarding compatibility information – see Section A, 2.2.

Formulation	Method	Dilution	Rate	Comments	Compatibility
Acetylcysteine					
Ampoule 2g/10mL	(C) IV infusion via a volumetric infusion pump.	**Paracetamol overdose:** dilute with G. Initially give 150mg/kg in 200mL over 15 minutes then 50mg/kg in 500mL over 4 hours, followed by 100mg/kg in 1L over 16 hours.		**Acute events that may accompany administration:** Anaphylactoid reactions may occur that appear to be dose related. Infusion should be temporarily stopped but can usually be restarted at a lower rate without further reaction. **pH:** 7 **Flush:** G or N/S **Sodium content:** 12.8mmol/10mL **Other comments:** The manufacturer also recommends other infusion fluids but G is preferable. A change in colour of solutions of acetylcysteine to light purple is insignificant.	
	IV bolus **(unlicensed practice precontrast)** preferably via central line.	Undiluted	3–5 minutes		

42

Formulation	Method	Dilution	Rate	Comments	Compatibility
Aciclovir (acyclovir)					
Vial 250mg, 500mg, 1g	(I) IV infusion	Reconstitute 250mg vial with 10mL and 500mg vial with 20mL of W or N/S (if supplied as a dry powder). Dilute to no more than 5mg/mL N/S. Fluid restriction: reconstitute vial as above and give centrally undiluted via a syringe pump (ensure that patient is well hydrated).	Minimum 1 hour	**Acute events that may accompany administration:** Extravasation may cause tissue damage; for management guidelines, see Section A, 7. **pH:** 11 **Flush:** N/S, G/S or H **Sodium content:** 1.1 mmol/250mg **Displacement:** Negligible **Other comments:** Use infusion within 12 hours. The reconstituted solution must not be refrigerated, therefore discard any remainder.	**Y-site compatible (but see Section A, 2.6):** ceftazidime, cefuroxime, cefotaxime, clindamycin, erythromycin, fluconazole, gentamicin, heparin, imipenem, magnesium sulphate, metronidazole, potassium chloride, propofol, tobramycin (both medicines in G), co-trimoxazole, vancomycin. **Incompatible:** dobutamine, dopamine, foscarnet, ondansetron, pethidine.

- For abbreviations used in the Table, see Section A, 2.4.
  e.g. (C) IV = continuous intravenous infusion; (I) IV = intermittent intravenous infusion.
- Prepare a fresh infusion every 24hours unless otherwise specified.
- Presume suitability as single-use only unless otherwise specified.
- Always check with additional reference sources regarding compatibility information – see Section A, 2.2.

Formulation	Method	Dilution	Rate	Comments	Compatibility
Addiphos					
Vial 20mL containing: phosphate 40mmol, potassium 30mmol	(I) IV infusion (unlicensed) into a central line via a volumetric infusion pump.	Dilute one vial in 500mL G. In fluid restriction can be diluted in 100mL.	Usual maximum rate 9mmol phosphate over 12 hours. Faster rates are used in ICU, i.e. one vial over 12–24 hours (local practice).	**Acute events that may accompany administration:** Oedema and hypotension, monitor blood pressure. Doses of phosphate exceeding 9mmol/12 hours may cause hypocalcaemia and metastatic calcification. Monitor calcium, phosphate, potassium, other electrolytes and renal function. Pain or phlebitis may occur during peripheral administration of solutions containing more than 30mmol/L potassium. **Flush:** G **Sodium content:** 30mmol/vial	Incompatible with calcium-containing fluids.
Adenosine					
Vial 6mg/2mL	IV bolus	May be diluted with N/S if necessary.	As quickly as possible (over 2 seconds).	**Acute events that may accompany administration:** Facial flushing, dyspnoea, tightness in chest. **ECG** monitoring normally required. Resuscitation equipment should be available. **pH:** 6.3–7.3 **Flush:** N/S **Sodium content:** Negligible **Other comments:** Inject as proximally as possible (into a central or large peripheral vein) and follow with a rapid N/S flush.	

Formulation	Method	Dilution	Rate	Comments	Compatibility
Adrenaline (epinephrine)					
Ampoule 1 in 1000 (1 mg/1 mL), 1 in 10000 (1 mg/10 mL)	(C) IV infusion via syringe or volumetric infusion pump. For emergency use: central line administration is recommended. If injected peripherally, the medicine must be flushed with at least 20 mL N/S.	Dilute 1 mg with 250 mL. N/S, G, G 10%, G/S or H. Unlicensed local practice (ICU) dilute 2, 4 or 8 mg to 50 mL with N/S or G. Undiluted solutions have been used (anecdotal).	Adjust rate according to response.	**Acute events that may accompany administration:** Arrhythmias – adrenaline infusions should be used in areas where appropriate cardiovascular monitoring is available (ICU, high dependency unit, etc.). Extravasation may cause tissue damage; for management guidelines see Section A, 7. **pH:** 2.5–3.6 **Do not flush:** Replace giving set **Other comments:** The IM route is preferred to S/C as it is more reliable. The prefilled syringes contain latex.	**Y-site compatible (but see Section A, 2.6):** atracurium, calcium gluconate, dobutamine, dopamine, fentanyl, furosemide, glyceryl trinitrate, heparin, midazolam, noradrenaline (norepinephrine) (in G/S or G only), pancuronium, potassium chloride, vecuronium. **Incompatible:** aminophylline, thiopental.
Min-I-Jet 1 in 10000 (1 mg/10 mL), 1 in 1000 (1 mg/1 mL)	IV bolus – emergency use.	Use Min-I-Jet or 1 mg/10 mL (1 in 10000) solution.			
	IM or S/C. See 'Other comments'.	0.5–1 mL of 1 in 1000 (1 mg/1 mL)			

- For abbreviations used in the Table, see Section A, 2.4.
  e.g. (C) IV = continuous intravenous infusion; (I) IV = intermittent intravenous infusion.
- Prepare a fresh infusion every 24 hours unless otherwise specified.
- Presume suitability as single-use only unless otherwise specified.
- Always check with additional reference sources regarding compatibility information – see Section A, 2.2.

45

Formulation	Method	Dilution	Rate	Comments	Compatibility
Alemtuzumab					
Vial 30mg	IV infusion	The required amount should be added to 100mL N/S or G. Invert bag gently to mix the solution.	120 minutes	**Acute events that may accompany administration:** May provoke hypersensitivity reactions, particularly with first dose, including fever chills, rigors, nausea and urticaria. These might be controlled by reducing the rate of infusion. More severe reactions have occurred eg. bronchospasm and hypotension. **pH:** 6.8–7.4 **Flush:** N/S or G **Displacement:** N/A **Sodium content:** 3.55 mg/mL **Other comments:** Premedication with paracetamol and IV chlorphenamine is recommended. Caution should be exercised in handling and preparing solution. The use of latex gloves and safety glasses is recommended to avoid exposure. Alemtuzumab is infused at a slower rate (over 8 hours) in a larger volume (500mL) for patients undergoing low-intensity BM/PBSC transplantations. Alemtuzumab is used in T-Deplete BM/PBSC transplantation; bags are incubated with alemtuzumab 30 minutes before reinfusion of cells.	Do not infuse with other medicines.

46

Formulation	Method	Dilution	Rate	Comments	Compatibility
Alfentanil					
Ampoule 1mg/2mL, 5mg/10mL, 5mg/1mL (for dilution)	IV bolus	May be diluted with N/S or G.	Minimum 30 seconds in spontaneously breathing patients.	**Acute events that may accompany administration:** Respiratory depression, apnoea and bradycardia. Hypotension may occur if administered too rapidly. Doses above 1 mg usually involve significant respiratory depression. **pH:** 4–6 **Flush:** N/S, G **Other comments:** *Anaesthesia:* adequate plasma levels will be achieved rapidly only if the infusion (0.5–1 micrograms/kg per minute) is preceded by a loading dose of 50–100 micrograms/kg given as a bolus or fast infusion over 10 minutes.	**Y-site compatible (but see Section A, 2.6):** atracurium, midazolam, propofol. **Incompatible:** alkaline agents, thiopental.
	(C) IV infusion via syringe pump. Use only in ventilated patients.	Dilute with N/S, G or H to a convenient volume.	See 'Other comments'.		

- For abbreviations used in the Table, see Section A, 2.4.
  e.g. (C) IV = continuous intravenous infusion; (I) IV = intermittent intravenous infusion.
- Prepare a fresh infusion every 24 hours unless otherwise specified.
- Presume suitability as single-use only unless otherwise specified.
- Always check with additional reference sources regarding compatibility information – see Section A, 2.2.

47

Formulation	Method	Dilution	Rate	Comments	Compatibility
Alprostadil					
(prostaglandin E₁) Ampoule 500 micrograms/ 1mL	(C) IV infusion via syringe pump. Via umbilical catheter.	Dilute with N/S or G usually to between 2 and 20 micrograms/ 1mL.	Variable according to indication. See package insert or specialist protocol for details.	**Acute events that may accompany administration:** Hypotension, monitor arterial pressure; decrease infusion rate immediately if pressure falls significantly. In neonates: apnoea, bradycardia; monitor blood pressure, heart rate, oxygen saturation and respiratory rate. **Do not flush:** Replace giving set **Sodium content:** Nil **Other comments:** Store unused ampoules in the refrigerator. If the reconstituted solution becomes hazy or the appearance of the container changes, discard the solution and replace the container. Add directly to the infusion solution, avoiding contact with the plastic walls of the infusion container.	
Alteplase					
Vial 20mg, 50mg	Initial IV bolus dose, then (I) IV infusion via syringe pump.	Reconstitute 20mg vial with 20mL of W and 50mg vial with 50mL W.	Variable according to indication. See package insert or specialist protocol for details.	**Acute events that may accompany administration:** Bleeding at injection site, intracerebral haemorrhage, nausea and vomiting. ECG and haemodynamic monitoring required. **pH:** 7.3 **Sodium content:** Nil **Flush:** N/S **Other comments:** A colourless to pale-yellow solution is produced. Foaming may occur, the bubbles will dissipate after standing for a few minutes. The reconstituted solution may be stored for up to 24 hours in the refrigerator and up to 8 hours at a temperature not exceeding 25°C.	**Y-site compatible (but see Section A, 2.6):** lidocaine. **Incompatible:** G, dobutamine, dopamine, glyceryl trinitrate, heparin.

Formulation	Method	Dilution	Rate	Comments	Compatibility
Amikacin					
Vial 100mg/2mL, 500mg/2mL	IV bolus (preferred method)	May be diluted with 10–20mL N/S, G	2–3 minutes	**pH:** 4.5 **Flush:** N/S, G **Sodium content:** 0.14mmol/100mg and 0.72mmol/500mg	Amikacin may be added to a metronidazole infusion bag. **Y-site compatible (but see Section A, 2.6):** aciclovir, amiodarone, fluconazole, foscarnet, midazolam, ondansetron. **Incompatible:** propofol, heparin, penicillins calcium gluconate, ranitidine.
	(I) IV infusion	Dilute to 2.5mg/1mL with N/S, G.	30 minutes		
	IM	Ready diluted			

- For abbreviations used in the Table, see Section A, 2.4.
  e.g. (C) IV = continuous intravenous infusion; (I) IV = intermittent intravenous infusion.
- Prepare a fresh infusion every 24hours unless otherwise specified.
- Presume suitability as single-use only unless otherwise specified.
- Always check with additional reference sources regarding compatibility information – see Section A, 2.2.

49

Formulation	Method	Dilution	Rate	Comments	Compatibility
Aminophylline					
Ampoule 250 mg/10 mL	(I) IV infusion (**initial loading dose**) via volumetric infusion pump	Dilute to 250 mL with N/S, G or G/S. Maximum concentration 25 mg/1 mL (administer centrally). **Paediatric information:** dilute to a concentration of 1 mg/1 mL.	**Adults:** usually 30 minutes (max. rate 25 mg/minute)	**Acute events that may accompany administration:** Tachycardia and hypotension, monitor heart rate and blood pressure. Arrhythmias and convulsions may occur if infusion rate is too fast. Extravasation may cause tissue damage; for management guidelines see Section A, 7. **pH:** 8.8–10 **Flush:** N/S, G or G/S **Other comments:** Plasma level monitoring is required. If the pH of the aminophylline solution falls below 8, crystals of theophylline will form. **Paediatric information:** Use a syringe or volumetric infusion pump.	**Y-site compatible (but see Section A, 2.6):** atracurium, ceftazidime, dexamethasone, dopamine, erythromycin, flucloxacillin, fluconazole, foscarnet, furosemide, glyceryl trinitrate, heparin, hydrocortisone sodium succinate, lidocaine, meropenem, metronidazole, netilmicin, pancuronium, phenylephrine, potassium chloride, propofol, piperacillin/tazobactam, ranitidine, terbutaline. **Incompatible:** adrenaline (epinephrine), amiodarone, bleomycin, cefotaxime, ciprofloxacin, clarithromycin, clindamycin, dobutamine, doxapram, doxorubicin, hydralazine, insulin (soluble), morphine, pethidine.
	(C) IV infusion (**maintenance dose**) via volumetric infusion pump	Dilute to 500 mL with N/S, G or G/S. Fluid restriction: maximum concentration 25 mg/1 mL (administer centrally). **Paediatric information:** dilute to a concentration of 1 mg/1 mL.	**Adults:** typically 0.5 mg/kg per hour		

Formulation	Method	Dilution	Rate	Comments	Compatibility
Amiodarone					
Ampoule 150mg/3mL	IV bolus – emergency use	Dilute each 150–300mg with 10–20mL G.	Minimum 3 minutes.	**Acute events that may accompany administration:** IV bolus: patient should be closely monitored, e.g. in an ICU because rapid administration may cause hypotension and circulatory collapse. Rapid administration may cause hypotension, anaphylactic shock, sweating, nausea and in patients with respiratory failure, bronchospasm and apnoea. **ECG** monitoring required. Thrombophlebitis at the site of infusion. Extravasation may cause tissue damage; for management guidelines see Section A, 7. **pH:** 3.5–4.5 **Flush:** G **Sodium content:** Nil **Other comments:** Very irritant, when repeated. For continuous infusion, administer via a central line. Avoid equipment containing the plasticiser di-2-ethylhexyphthalate (DEHP) (see BNF).	**Y-site compatible (but see Section A, 2.6):** amikacin, bretylium, clarithromycin, clindamycin, dobutamine, dopamine, erythromycin, gentamicin, glyceryl trinitrate, insulin (soluble), isoprenaline, lidocaine, metronidazole, midazolam, noradrenaline (norepinephrine), phenylephrine, potassium chloride, procainamide, streptokinase, vancomycin. **Incompatible:** aminophylline, flucloxacillin, furosemide, heparin, N/S, sodium bicarbonate.
	(I) IV infusion (loading dose). Administration via a volumetric infusion pump is preferred as amiodarone may reduce drop size. See 'Other comments'.	Dilute loading dose (5mg/kg) in 250mL G. Dilution to a concentration of less than 600 micrograms/mL is unstable. Solutions of <300mg/ 500mL G should not be used.	Over 20 minutes to 2 hours.		
	(C) IV infusion (maintenance dose) via volumetric infusion pump. See 'Other comments'.	Dilute dose (15mg/kg, max. 1200mg) in 500mL G. In fluid restriction: up to 900mg in 50mL G centrally (anecdotal).	24 hours.		

- For abbreviations used in the Table, see Section A, 2.4.
  e.g. (C) IV = continuous intravenous infusion; (I) IV = intermittent intravenous infusion.
- Prepare a fresh infusion every 24hours unless otherwise specified.
- Presume suitability as single-use only unless otherwise specified.
- Always check with additional reference sources regarding compatibility information – see Section A, 2.2.

Formulation	Method	Dilution	Rate	Comments	Compatibility
Amoxicillin					
Vial 250 mg, 500 mg	IV bolus (preferred method)	Reconstitute 250 mg with 5 mL W and 500 mg with 10 mL W.	3–4 minutes	**pH:** 8.6–8.8 **Flush:** N/S **Sodium content:** 3.2 mmol/1 g **Displacement:** 0.2 mL/250 mg (0.4 mL/500 mg). Add 4.8 mL diluent to 250 mg vial to give a concentration of 50 mg in 1 mL or 9.8 mL diluent to 250 mg vial to give a concentration of 25 mg in 1 mL. **Other comments:** Use infusion within 8 hours. A transient pink coloration or slight opalescence may appear during reconstitution. Reconstituted solutions may be a pale straw colour.	**Incompatible:** aminoglycosides, ciprofloxacin.
	(I) IV infusion	Reconstitute as above then dilute with 50–100 mL N/S.	30–60 minutes		
	IM	Reconstitute 250 mg with 1.5 mL W and 500 mg with 2.5 mL W. Substitute lidocaine 1% for W if pain is a problem.			

52

Formulation	Method	Dilution	Rate	Comments	Compatibility
Amphotericin (Fungizone)					
Vial 50mg (50000 units)	(Fungizone) (I) IV infusion via a volumetric infusion pump	Reconstitute vial with 10ml W to give a 5mg/1mL solution. See 'Other comments' for use of 'phosphate buffer'. Dilute volume required with 50 times as much buffered G to produce a maximum concentration of 10mg/100mL for peripheral administration. For central administration: dilutions up to 40mg/100mL have been used (unlicensed).	2–4 hours. Rarely up to 6 hours. The CSM advise administration of a test dose on initiation of therapy. Typically administer 1mg over 20–30 minutes and observe the patient for a furthers 30 minutes.	**Acute events that may accompany administration: Rapid infusion** may increase side effects. Peripheral administration may cause local venous pain at the injection site with phlebitis and thrombophlebitis. This may be relieved by the addition of heparin 500–1000 units to the infusion bag. Fever (sometimes with shaking chills) may be relieved by adding pethidine 50mg to the infusion bag (as long as heparin has not been added due to lack of compatibility data). Other side effects include headache and vomiting. **pH:** 5.7 **Flush:** With G before and after administration. **Sodium content:** Negligible **Displacement:** Negligible **Other comments:** The manufacturers recommend that the pH of G must exceed 4.2 to prevent precipitation. To ensure this, add phosphate buffer to G before amphotericin is added. The phosphate buffer label should state the volume of phosphate to be added to the amphotericin. To reduce nephrotoxicity, prehydrate with N/S 1L.	May be mixed in an infusion bag with pethidine (local practice) *or* heparin. **Y-site compatible (but see Section A, 2.6):** heparin, sodium bicarbonate. **Incompatible:** N/S, benzylpenicillin, calcium salts, cimetidine, dobutamine, dopamine, fluconazole, foscarnet, gentamicin, meropenem, ondansetron, piperacillin/ tazobactam, potassium chloride, propofol, ranitidine.

- For abbreviations used in the Table, see Section A, 2.4.
  e.g. (C) IV = continuous intravenous infusion; (I) IV = intermittent intravenous infusion.
- Prepare a fresh infusion every 24hours unless otherwise specified.
- Presume suitability as single-use only unless otherwise specified.
- Always check with additional reference sources regarding compatibility information – see Section A, 2.2.

Formulation	Method	Dilution	Rate	Comments	Compatibility
Amphotericin lipid complex (Abelcet)					
Vial 100 mg/20 mL	(I) IV Infusion via a volumetric infusion pump	Allow suspension to reach room temperature, shake gently to ensure no yellow sediment. Withdraw the required dose into a syringe and add to G through the 5 µm filter needle provided (use a fresh needle for each syringe) to produce a final concentration of 1 mg/mL. In fluid-restricted patients or children dilute to 2 mg/mL with G.	2.5 mg/kg per hour. For test dose see 'Other comments'.	**Acute events that may accompany administration:** Apnoea. **pH:** 5–7 (undiluted) **Flush:** before and after administration with G. **Sodium content:** 3.13 mmol/vial **Other comments:** It is advisable to administer a test dose on initiation of therapy even if the patient had previously tolerated an alternative amphotericin formulation. Typically 1 mL (5 mg) in 100 mL G should be infused IV over 15 minute.	**Incompatible:** N/S. Do not mix with other medicines or fluids.

Formulation	Method	Dilution	Rate	Comments	Compatibility
Amphotericin liposomal (AmBisome)					
Vial 50mg	(I) IV infusion	Add 12ml W to 50mg vial and shake vigorously for at least 15 seconds. Resulting amphotericin concentration 4mg/1mL. Dilute dose required through the 5 µm filter provided with between 1 and 19 parts of G by volume, to give a final concentration of between 0.2mg/1mL and 2mg/1mL.	30–60 minutes. For test dose see 'Other comments'.	**pH:** 5–6 **Flush:** Before and after administration with G. **Sodium content:** <0.5mmol/vial **Other comments:** A 50mg vial contains about 900mg sucrose. It is advisable to administer a test dose on initiation of therapy even if the patient had previously tolerated an alternative amphotericin formulation. A small dose (i.e. 1mg) should be infused over about 10 minutes and the patient carefully observed for 30 minutes. Protect infusion from light. Reconstituted product may be stored for up to 24 hours in the refrigerator.	**Incompatible:** N/S. Do not mix with other medicines or fluids.

- For abbreviations used in the Table, see Section A, 2.4.
  e.g. (C) IV = continuous intravenous infusion; (I) IV = intermittent intravenous infusion.
- Prepare a fresh infusion every 24 hours unless otherwise specified.
- Presume suitability as single-use only unless otherwise specified.
- Always check with additional reference sources regarding compatibility information – see Section A, 2.2.

Formulation	Method	Dilution	Rate	Comments	Compatibility
Aprotinin					
Vial 500000 kallikrein inactivator units (KIU)/ 50mL	IV bolus (initial loading dose)	Provided ready diluted. May be diluted with N/S, G or G/S.	Maximum rate 10mL of original solution/minute. For test dose see 'Other comments'.	**Acute events that may accompany administration:** Hypersensitivity reactions. Peripheral administration may occasionally cause thrombophlebitis. **pH:** 5–7 **Flush:** N/S, G **Sodium content:** 7.7 mmol/50mL **Other comments:** Patient should be supine for administration. The manufacturers recommend that an initial 1 ml loading dose should be infused slowly to test for allergic reactions. If contents of vial are cloudy do not use.	Do not infuse with other medicines.
	(C) IV infusion	As above.	20–50mL of original solution/hour. For test dose see 'Other comments'.		

Formulation	Method	Dilution	Rate	Comments	Compatibility
Atenolol					
Vial 5 mg/10 mL	IV bolus	May be diluted with N/S, G or G/S.	Max. rate 1 mg/minute	**Acute events that may accompany administration:** Severe bradycardia and hypotension, monitor heart rate and blood pressure. Can cause conduction defects, monitor **ECG.** If infused too quickly there is a higher incidence of the above effects. **pH:** 5.5–6.5 **Flush:** N/S, G or G/S	
	(I) IV infusion via volumetric infusion pump	Dilute with N/S, G or G/S.	20 minutes		
Atosiban					
Vial 6. 6.75 mg/ 0.9 mL, 37.5 mg/5 mL vial	IV bolus (loading dose first)	Ready diluted.	6.75 mg over 1 minute.	**Acute events that may accompany administration:** Allergic reaction, injection site reaction, nausea and vomiting, hyperglycaemia, headache, dizziness, tachycardia, hypotension. **Sodium content:** Nil **pH:** 4.1–4.9 **Flush:** N/S **Other comments:** Use diluted medicine within 24 hours of preparation.	Do not infuse with other medicines
	(C) IV infusion (following IV bolus)	Withdraw and discard 10 mL from a 100 mL bag of N/S or G and add 10 mL atosiban 7.5 mg/mL to provide 75 mg in 100 mL.	Run at 24 mL/hour for 3 hours then 8 mL/hour for up to 45 hours. Maximum 48 hours therapy.		

- For abbreviations used in the Table, see Section A, 2.4.
  e.g. (C) IV = continuous intravenous infusion; (I) IV = intermittent intravenous infusion.
- Prepare a fresh infusion every 24 hours unless otherwise specified.
- Presume suitability as single-use only unless otherwise specified.
- Always check with additional reference sources regarding compatibility information – see Section A, 2.2.

Formulation	Method	Dilution	Rate	Comments	Compatibility
Atracurium					
Ampoule 25 mg/2.5 mL, 50 mg/5 mL, 250 mg/25 mL	IV bolus	May be administered undiluted or may be diluted with G, G/S or N/S.	1 minute	**Acute events that may accompany administration:** Histamine release may produce flushing and rarely bronchospasm. **pH:** 3.5 **Flush:** N/S	**Y-site compatible (but see Section A, 2.6):** alfentanil, co-trimoxazole (both medicines in G), dobutamine, dopamine, fentanyl, gentamicin, glyceryl trinitrate, heparin, isoprenaline, midazolam, morphine, potassium chloride, sodium nitroprusside. **Incompatible:** alkaline agents, aminophylline, propofol, thiopental.
	(C) IV infusion via syringe pump	May be administered undiluted or can be diluted with G, G/S or N/S.	300–600 micrograms/kg per hour		
Atropine					
Ampoule 600 micro-grams/1 mL, Min-I-Jet 1 mg/10 mL, Pre-filled syringe 3 mg/10 mL	IV bolus	Ready diluted.	Give rapidly as slow IV administration may cause paradoxical slowing of the heart	**Acute events that may accompany administration:** Arrhythmias and paradoxical slowing of the heart, monitor **ECG** if feasible. Extravasation may cause tissue damage; for management guidelines, see Section A, 7. **pH:** 3–4.5 **Flush:** N/S	**Y-site compatible (but see Section A, 2.6):** dobutamine, furosemide, heparin, meropenem, midazolam, morphine, propofol, potassium chloride. **Incompatible:** alkaline agents including noradrenaline (norepinephrine), sodium bicarbonate.
	S/C or IM				

Formulation	Method	Dilution	Rate	Comments	Compatibility
Augmentin					
	See Co-amoxiclav				
Azathioprine					
Vial 50mg	(I) IV infusion (preferred method) via volumetric infusion or syringe pump	**Handle as for cytotoxic medicines** Reconstitute with a minimum of 5–15mL W and then dilute with 20–200mL N/S or G/S.	30–60 minutes	**Acute events that may accompany administration:** Extravasation may cause tissue damage; for management guidelines, see Section A, 7. **pH:** 10–12 (pH 8–9.5 when diluted with N/S or G/S) **Flush:** N/S or G **Sodium content:** 0.2mmol/vial **Displacement:** Negligible **Other comments:** Discard if any turbidity or crystallisation occurs.	Do not infuse with other medicines.
	IV bolus into a Y-site of a fast flowing N/S or G drip. Flush with at least 50mL N/S or G/S as very irritant	**Handle as for cytotoxic medicines** Reconstitute with a minimum of 5–15mL W.	Usually 3–5 minutes. Min. 1 minute		

• For abbreviations used in the Table, see Section A, 2.4.
e.g. (C) IV = continuous intravenous infusion; (I) IV = intermittent intravenous infusion.
• Prepare a fresh infusion every 24hours unless otherwise specified.
• Presume suitability as single-use only unless otherwise specified.
• Always check with additional reference sources regarding compatibility information – see Section A, 2.2.

Formulation	Method	Dilution	Rate	Comments	Compatibility
Benzylpenicillin					
Vial 600mg	IV bolus (preferred method)	Reconstitute each 600mg with 4–10mL W, N/S or G.	**Adults:** 3–5 minutes. Max. rate 300mg/minute	**Acute events that may accompany administration:** Rapid administration may cause CNS irritation leading to convulsions. Anaphylaxis. **pH:** 6.8 **Flush:** N/S or G **Sodium content:** 1.68mmol/vial **Displacement:** 0.4mL/600mg Add 3.6mL diluent to 600mg vial to give a concentration of 600mg/4mL.	**Y-site compatible (but see Section A, 2.6):** heparin. **Incompatible:** amphotericin, flucloxacillin, aminoglycosides, e.g. gentamicin, tranexamic acid.
	(I) IV infusion	Reconstitute as above then dilute each 600mg with a minimum of 10mL N/S or G (suggested volume 100mL).	30–60 minutes		
	IM	Reconstitute each 600mg with 1.6mL W.			

Formulation	Method	Dilution	Rate	Comments	Compatibility
Bumetanide					
Ampoule 1 mg/2 mL, 2 mg/4 mL, 5 mg/10 mL	IV bolus (for doses up to 2 mg)	May be diluted with N/S or G if necessary. May be given undiluted.	Max. rate 1 mg/minute	**Acute events that may accompany administration:** Hypotension, monitor blood pressure. Myalgia is common if doses above 2 mg are given as a bolus. **pH:** 6.8–7.8 **Flush:** N/S **Sodium content:** Negligible **Other comments:** Discard if cloudiness develops.	**Y-site compatible (but see Section A, 2.6):** clarithromycin, morphine, pethidine, propofol, piperacillin/tazobactam. **Incompatible:** dobutamine, midazolam.
	(I) IV infusion (for doses above 2 mg)	Dilute to a suitable volume with G, N/S or G/S to a maximum concentration of 1 mg in 10 mL.	30 minutes		
	IM.	Ready diluted.			

- For abbreviations used in the Table, see Section A, 2.4.
  e.g. (C) IV = continuous intravenous infusion; (I) IV = intermittent intravenous infusion.
- Prepare a fresh infusion every 24 hours unless otherwise specified.
- Presume suitability as single-use only unless otherwise specified.
- Always check with additional reference sources regarding compatibility information – see Section A, 2.2.

61

Formulation	Method	Dilution	Rate	Comments	Compatibility
Buprenorphine					
Ampoule 300 micrograms/1 mL	IV bolus	May be diluted with N/S or G	At least 2 minutes	**Acute events that may accompany administration:** Hypotension and respiratory depression, monitor blood pressure and respiration rate. Sedation, monitor sedation scores. Extravasation may cause tissue damage; for management guidelines see Section A, 7. **pH:** 3.5–5.5 **Flush:** N/S **Sodium content:** Nil	**Y-site compatible (but see Section A, 2.6):** atropine. **Incompatible:** diazepam, lorazepam.
	Deep IM injection	Ready diluted.			

Formulation	Method	Dilution	Rate	Comments	Compatibility
Caffeine citrate					
Ampoule 10mg/1mL	(I) IV infusion (loading dose)	Dilute with N/S or G.	20 minutes	**Acute events that may accompany administration:** Injection site reactions. **pH:** 2–3.5 **Flush:** N/S or G **Sodium content:** Nil **Other comments:** As a result of acidity of caffeine, it is preferable to administer centrally. Can monitor levels if signs of toxicity. Caffeine should be prescribed as the citrate to avoid confusion with the base which has a different dose.	Do not infuse with other medicines.
	IV bolus (maintenance dose)	Undiluted.	5 minutes		

- For abbreviations used in the Table, see Section A, 2.4.
  e.g. (C) IV = continuous intravenous infusion; (I) IV = intermittent intravenous infusion.
- Prepare a fresh infusion every 24hours unless otherwise specified.
- Presume suitability as single-use only unless otherwise specified.
- Always check with additional reference sources regarding compatibility information – see Section A, 2.2.

Formulation	Method	Dilution	Rate	Comments	Compatibility
Calcium chloride					
Min-I-Jet 10% 10mL containing 6.8mmol calcium/10mL. Calcium chloride 10mmol in 10mL ampoule	IV bolus – emergency use	Ready diluted.		**Acute events that may accompany administration:** Rapid IV administration may cause vasodilatation, decreased blood pressure, bradycardia, cardiac arrhythmias, syncope and cardiac arrest. Very irritant; always administer slowly. Extravasation may cause tissue damage; for management guidelines see Section A, 7. **pH:** 5.5–7.5 **Flush:** G, G/S, N/S	**Compatibility/ Incompatibility:** see calcium gluconate.
Calcium folinate					
See Folinic acid					

Formulation	Method	Dilution	Rate	Comments	Compatibility
Calcium gluconate					
Ampoule 10%, 10 mL containing 2.2 mmol calcium/10 mL	IV bolus – emergency use	Ready diluted.	**Adults:** max. rate 0.44 mmol calcium (2 mL of 10%)/minute **Neonates:** see cBNF for advice	**Acute events that may accompany administration:** Rapid IV administration may cause vasodilation, decreased blood pressure, bradycardia, cardiac arrhythmias, syncope and cardiac arrest. Extravasation may cause tissue damage; for management guidelines see Section A, 7. **pH:** 6–8 **Flush:** N/S	**Y-site compatible (but see Section A, 2.6):** amikacin, dobutamine, heparin, lidocaine, noradrenaline (norepinephrine), potassium chloride. **Incompatible:** amphotericin, bicarbonates, carbonates, citrates, clindamycin, fluconazole, hydrocortisone sodium succinate, sulphates, pamidronate, phosphates, tartrates.
	(I) IV or (C) IV infusion	Dilute with N/S, G or G/S. Fluid restriction: can be infused undiluted.			

- For abbreviations used in the Table, see Section A, 2.4.
  e.g. (C) IV = continuous intravenous infusion; (I) IV = intermittent intravenous infusion.
- Prepare a fresh infusion every 24 hours unless otherwise specified.
- Presume suitability as single-use only unless otherwise specified.
- Always check with additional reference sources regarding compatibility information – see Section A, 2.2.

Formulation	Method	Dilution	Rate	Comments	Compatibility
Caspofungin					
Vials 70mg and 50mg	(I) IV infusion	70mg vial: reconstitute with 10.5mL W producing a solution of 7mg/mL. Add 10mL of the reconstituted caspofungin to 250mL N/S. 50mg vial: reconstitute with 10.5mL W producing a solution of 5mg/mL. Add 10mL of the reconstituted caspofungin to 250mL N/S.	60 minutes	**Acute events that may accompany administration:** Fever and phlebitis. **pH:** 6.6 **Flush:** N/S **Sodium content:** 50mg vial – 0.028mmol/mL, 70mg vial – 0.04mmol/mL **Other comments:** 50mg doses (but not 70mg) may be administered in 100mL N/S if required in fluid restriction.	Caspofungin is not stable in diluents containing G. Do not mix or co-infuse caspofungin with other medicinal products, as there are no compatibility data available.

Formulation	Method	Dilution	Rate	Comments	Compatibility
Cefotaxime					
Vial 500mg, 1g, 2g	IV bolus (preferred method)	Reconstitute 500mg with 2mL, 1g with 4mL and 2g with 10mL W.	3–5 minutes	**pH:** 4.5–6.5 **Flush:** N/S or G **Sodium content:** 2.09mmol/1g **Displacement:** 0.2mL/500mg vial, 0.5mL/1g vial, 1.2mL/2g vial. Add 1.8mL of diluent to 500mg vial to give a concentration of 500mg in 2mL (250mg in 1mL). **Other comments:** Reconstituted cefotaxime forms a straw-coloured solution. Variations in the intensity of colour do not indicate changes in potency or safety.	Cefotaxime may be added to a metronidazole infusion bag. **Y-site compatible (but see Section A, 2.6):** aciclovir, heparin, morphine, midazolam, pethidine, propofol. **Incompatible:** alkaline agents, aminoglycosides, aminophylline, fluconazole.
	(I) IV infusion	Reconstitute as above, then dilute each 1g or 2g with 40–100mL N/S, G, G/S or H.	20–60 minutes		
	IM	Reconstitute 500mg with 2mL, 1g with 4mL and 2g with 10mL W. Doses of 2g should be divided and administered at different sites.			

- For abbreviations used in the Table, see Section A, 2.4.
  e.g. (C) IV = continuous intravenous infusion; (I) IV = intermittent intravenous infusion.
- Prepare a fresh infusion every 24 hours unless otherwise specified.
- Presume suitability as single-use only unless otherwise specified.
- Always check with additional reference sources regarding compatibility information – see Section A, 2.2.

67

Formulation	Method	Dilution	Rate	Comments	Compatibility
Ceftazidime					
Vial 250 mg, 500 mg, 1 g, 2 g	IV bolus (preferred method) Max. dose 2 g	Reconstitute 250 mg with a minimum of 2.5 mL, 500 mg with 5 mL, 1 g and 2 g with 10 mL W, N/S or G.	3–5 minutes	**pH:** 5–8 **Flush:** N/S, G, G/S or Hep/S **Sodium content:** 2.3 mmol/1 g **Displacement:** 0.25 mL/250 mg Add 2.25 mL of diluent to 250 mg vial to give a concentration of 250 mg/2.5 mL (100 mg in 1 mL).	**Y-site compatible (but see Section A, 2.6):** aciclovir, heparin, hydrocortisone sodium succinate, potassium chloride. **Incompatible:** aminoglycosides, fluconazole, sodium bicarbonate.
	(I) IV infusion	Reconstitute as above then dilute to 50–100 mL with N/S, G or G/S.	Max. 30 minutes		
	Deep IM	Reconstitute 250 mg with 1 mL W, 500 mg with 1.5 mL W and 1 g with 3 mL W; 2 g not recommended.			

68

Formulation	Method	Dilution	Rate	Comments	Compatibility
Ceftriaxone					
Vials 250 mg, 1 g, 2 g	IV bolus (preferred for 1 g dose)	**1 g vial** IV bolus: dissolve in 10 mL W.	2–4 minutes	**Acute events that may accompany administration:** Pain/discomfort at site of IM injection, Local phlebitis. **pH:** 6.7 **Flush:** N/S **Sodium content:** 3.6 mmol/1 g **Displacement:** 0.8 mL/1 g, 1.03 mL/2 g **Other comments:** Reconstituted solutions with water for injection are a pale-yellow to amber colour. Do not use if particles present.	**Additive compatibility:** aminophylline, clindamycin phosphate, theophylline. **Y-site compatibility:** amphotericin B, pentamidine. **Incompatible:** calcium-containing solutions (e.g. H, Ringer's), amscarine, vancomycin, fluconazole, aminoglycosides, labetalol, linezolid.
	(I) IV infusion (preferred for 2 g dose)	**2 g vial** (I) IV infusion: dissolve in 40 mL N/S or G.	30 minutes		
	Deep IM injection	**1 g vial:** dissolve in 3.5 mL 1% lidocaine hydrochloride injection. **2 g vial:** dissolve in 7 mL 1% lidocaine hydrochloride injection.	IM injection: doses greater than 1 g should be given in more than one site		

- For abbreviations used in the Table, see Section A, 2.4.
  e.g. (C) IV = continuous intravenous infusion; (I) IV = intermittent intravenous infusion.
- Prepare a fresh infusion every 24 hours unless otherwise specified.
- Presume suitability as single-use only unless otherwise specified.
- Always check with additional reference sources regarding compatibility information – see Section A, 2.2.

Formulation	Method	Dilution	Rate	Comments	Compatibility
Cefuroxime					
Vial 250 mg, 750 mg, 1.5 g	IV bolus (preferred method)	Reconstitute 250 mg with at least 2 mL W, 750 mg with 6 mL W and 1.5 g with 15 mL W. May be diluted with N/S, G or G/S.	3–5 minutes	**pH:** 6–8.5 **Flush:** N/S, G or G/S **Sodium content:** 1.8 mmol/750 mg **Displacement:** 0.18 mL/250 mg vial Add 2.32 mL of diluent to 250 mg vial to give a concentration of 250 mg/2.5 mL (100 mg in 1 mL).	Cefuroxime may be added to a metronidazole infusion bag. **Y-site compatible (but see Section A, 2.6):** aciclovir, foscarnet, heparin, morphine. **Incompatible:** aminoglycosides, doxapram, fluconazole, sodium bicarbonate.
	(I) IV infusion	Reconstitute as above then dilute to 50–100 mL with N/S, G, or H.	Maximum 30 minutes		
	IM	Reconstitute 250 mg with 1 mL W, 750 mg with 3 mL W (1.5 g for IV administration only).			

Formulation	Method	Dilution	Rate	Comments	Compatibility
Chloramphenicol sodium succinate					
Vial 1 g	IV bolus	Reconstitute vial with 9.2 mL W, N/S or G (100 mg/1 mL). Other dilutions may be used (see package insert for details). Suggested max. concentration 100 mg/1 mL.	1 minute	**Acute events that may accompany administration:** Diarrhoea, optic neuritis and headache. Pain at injection site. **pH:** 6.4–7 **Flush:** N/S **Sodium content:** 3.14 mmol/1 g **Displacement:** 0.8 mL/1 g vial Add 9.2 mL of diluent to 1 g vial to give a concentration of 1 g/10 mL (100 mg in 1 mL). **Other comments:** Absorption from the IM route may be slow and unpredictable.	**Y-site compatible (but see Section A, 2.6):** aciclovir, dopamine, foscarnet, heparin, hydrocortisone sodium succinate, morphine. **Incompatible:** fluconazole, pethidine, phenothiazines, e.g. prochlorperazine, tetracyclines.
	(I) IV infusion	Reconstitute as above then dilute with N/S, G or G/S.			
	IM See 'Other comments'	Reconstitute vial with 1.7 mL W, N/S or G (400 mg/1 mL). Other dilutions may be used (see package insert for details).			

- For abbreviations used in the Table, see Section A, 2.4.
  e.g. (C) IV = continuous intravenous infusion; (I) IV = intermittent intravenous infusion.
- Prepare a fresh infusion every 24 hours unless otherwise specified.
- Presume suitability as single-use only unless otherwise specified.
- Always check with additional reference sources regarding compatibility information – see Section A, 2.2.

71

Formulation	Method	Dilution	Rate	Comments	Compatibility
Chloroquine sulphate					
Ampoule 272.5 mg/5 mL (200 mg/5 mL chloroquine base)	(C) IV infusion (preferred method)	Dilute with N/S.		**Acute events that may accompany administration:** Rapid IV infusion may result in cardiovascular toxicity and other symptoms of acute overdose e.g. hypotension and arrhythmias. **pH:** 4–5.5 **Flush:** N/S	Do not infuse with other medicines.
	IM (should be avoided in children)	Ready diluted.			
	S/C	Ready diluted.			
Chlorphenamine					
Ampoule 10 mg/1 mL	IV bolus	Dilute with 5–10 mL N/S, W (or patient's own blood).	Min. 1 minute	**Acute events that may accompany administration:** Rapid injection may cause transitory hypotension or CNS stimulation. **pH:** 4–5.2 **Flush:** N/S	Do not administer with other medicines.
	IM or S/C	Ready diluted.			

Formulation	Method	Dilution	Rate	Comments	Compatibility
Ciclosporin					
Ampoule 50 mg/1 mL, 250 mg/5 mL	(I) IV infusion via syringe or volumetric infusion pump	Dilute to between 1 in 20 and 1 in 100 by volume with N/S or G, i.e. 1 mL (50 mg) in 20–100 mL. Fluid restriction: no more concentrated than 2.5 mg/mL.	2–6 hours. Administration rates may vary in accordance with trial protocols or local practice (see 'Other comments').	**Acute events that may accompany administration:** Anaphylactic reactions; continuously observe patient for first 30 minute after initiation of infusion and subsequently monitor patient frequently. **pH:** 6–7 **Flush:** N/S **Other comments:** Not to be used with PVC equipment. Protect ampoules from light. Prepared infusions do not need to be protected from light. Plasma level monitoring is required.	

- For abbreviations used in the Table, see Section A, 2.4.
  e.g. (C) IV = continuous intravenous infusion; (I) IV = intermittent intravenous infusion.
- Prepare a fresh infusion every 24 hours unless otherwise specified.
- Presume suitability as single-use only unless otherwise specified.
- Always check with additional reference sources regarding compatibility information – see Section A, 2.2.

Formulation	Method	Dilution	Rate	Comments	Compatibility
Cidofovir					
Vial 375 mg/5 mL	(I) IV infusion	Dilute in 100 mL N/S.	60 minutes	**Acute events that may accompany administration:** To minimise nephrotoxicity: give oral probenecid 2 g 3 hours before cidofovir infusion followed by probenecid 1 g at 2 hours and 1 g at 8 hours after the end of cidofovir infusion. Prehydration with N/S IV infusion 1000 mL over 1 hour immediately before cidofovir infusion. **pH:** 7.4 **Flush:** N/S **Other comments:** Adequate precautions including the use of appropriate safety equipment are recommended for preparation, administration and disposal. Personnel preparing the reconstituted solution should wear surgical gloves, safety glasses and a closed front surgical-type gown with knit cuffs. If cidofovir contacts the skin, wash membranes and flush thoroughly with water.	No data are available to support the addition of other medicinal products or supplements to the recommended admixture for intravenous infusion. Compatibility with Ringer's, H or bacteriostatic infusion fluids has not been evaluated.

Formulation	Method	Dilution	Rate	Comments	Compatibility
Cimetidine					
Ampoule 200mg/2mL	(I) IV infusion (preferred method). See 'Other comments'	Dilute with N/S or G usually to 100mL.	30–60 minutes	**Acute events that may accompany administration:** Cardiac arrhythmias, monitor blood pressure and heart rate. Rapid IV administration may cause arrhythmias. **pH:** 4–6 **Flush:** N/S or G **Other comments:** (I) IV infusion must be used for doses over 200mg or if there is cardiovascular impairment.	**Incompatible:** amphotericin
	IV bolus See 'Other comments'	Dilute with 20mL N/S.	5 minutes		
	(C) IV infusion	Dilute with N/S or G to a convenient volume.	50–100mg/hour		
	IM	Ready diluted.			

- For abbreviations used in the Table, see Section A, 2.4.
  e.g. (C) IV = continuous intravenous infusion; (I) IV = intermittent intravenous infusion.
- Prepare a fresh infusion every 24hours unless otherwise specified.
- Presume suitability as single-use only unless otherwise specified.
- Always check with additional reference sources regarding compatibility information – see Section A, 2.2.

Formulation	Method	Dilution	Rate	Comments	Compatibility
Ciprofloxacin					
Vial 100mg/50mL. Infusion bag 200mg/100mL, 400mg/200mL	(I) IV infusion	Ready diluted.	100–200mg over 30–60 minutes; 400mg over 60 minutes	**pH:** 3.9–4.5 **Flush:** N/S **Sodium content:** 15.4mmol/100mL	**Y-site compatible (but see Section A, 2.6):** G, N/S, G/S, clarithromycin, dobutamine, dopamine, digoxin, gentamicin, lidocaine, metronidazole, midazolam, potassium chloride, tobramycin. **Incompatible:** aminophylline, clindamycin, dexamethasone, flucloxacillin, furosemide, heparin, hydrocortisone sodium succinate, methylprednisolone, penicillins, phenytoin, propofol, teicoplanin.

Formulation	Method	Dilution	Rate	Comments	Compatibility
Clarithromycin					
Vial 500mg	(I) IV infusion in large proximal vein	Reconstitute each vial with 10mL W, producing a solution containing 50mg/1mL. Dilute resultant solution with N/S, G or H to produce a final solution of approximately 2mg/1mL (e.g. 500mg in 250mL). In fluid restriction: 5mg/1mL via central line.	60 minutes	**Acute events that may accompany administration:** Phlebitis, tenderness and inflammation at injection site. Rapid infusion may cause arrhythmias. **pH:** 5 (in N/S) **Flush:** N/S or G **Sodium content:** Negligible **Displacement value:** 0.4mL/500mg vial BUT each vial actually contains 520mg, so when 10mL withdrawn the dose given will be 500mg. **Other comments:** Reconstituted solution is stable for 24 hours from 5–25°C. The final diluted product (2mg in 1mL) should be used within 6 hours if stored at room temperature or within 24 hours if refrigerated.	Do not infuse with other medicines.

- For abbreviations used in the Table, see Section A, 2.4.
  e.g. (C) IV = continuous intravenous infusion; (I) IV = intermittent intravenous infusion.
- Prepare a fresh infusion every 24 hours unless otherwise specified.
- Presume suitability as single-use only unless otherwise specified.
- Always check with additional reference sources regarding compatibility information – see Section A, 2.2.

77

Formulation	Method	Dilution	Rate	Comments	Compatibility
Clindamycin					
Ampoule 300 mg/2 mL, 600 mg/4 mL	(I) IV infusion (maximum dose 1.2 g)	Dilute to a concentration of 6 mg/1 mL with G or N/S (300 mg in 50 mL of G or N/S) Max. concentration 18 mg/1 mL.	1.2 g over at least 60 minutes	**Acute events that may accompany administration:** Thrombophlebitis, erythema, pain and swelling. Rare cases of cardiopulmonary arrest and hypotension following too rapid IV administration. **pH:** 5.5–7 **Flush:** N/S	**Y-site compatible (but see Section A, 2.6):** amiodarone, heparin sodium, foscarnet, midazolam, morphine, pethidine, piperacillin/ tazobactam, potassium chloride, propofol, zidovudine (both medicines in G). **Incompatible:** aminophylline, calcium salts, fluconazole, magnesium sulphate, phenytoin.
	(C) IV infusion (doses above 1.2 g)	Seek advice.			
	IM (maximum 600 mg)	Ready diluted.			

Formulation	Method	Dilution	Rate	Comments	Compatibility
Clonazepam					
Ampoule 1 mg/1 mL	IV bolus – emergency use into large vein of the antecubital fossa	Immediately before use dilute each 1 mg in 1 mL W, to produce a 1 mg in 2 mL solution.	Maximum rate 1 mg per 30 seconds	**Acute events that may accompany administration:** Hypotension, apnoea, monitor blood pressure and respiratory function. Salivary or bronchial hypersecretion. Extravasation may cause tissue damage; for management guidelines see Section A, 7. **pH:** 3.4–4.3 **Flush:** N/S **Sodium content:** Nil **Other comments:** IV infusion of clonazepam is potentially hazardous especially if prolonged. Close and constant observation required, preferably in centres with ITU facilities. Contains benzyl alcohol and propylene glycol up to 1 mL. Discard unused infusion after 12 hours.	
	(I) IV infusion via volumetric infusion pump	Dilute up to 3 mg in 250 mL G, G 10%, G/S or N/S.	Ideally should be infused over no longer than 2 hours. See 'Other comments'.		

- For abbreviations used in the Table, see Section A, 2.4.
  e.g. (C) IV = continuous intravenous infusion; (I) IV = intermittent intravenous infusion.
- Prepare a fresh infusion every 24 hours unless otherwise specified.
- Presume suitability as single-use only unless otherwise specified.
- Always check with additional reference sources regarding compatibility information – see Section A, 2.2.

Formulation	Method	Dilution	Rate	Comments	Compatibility
Clonidine					
Ampoule 150 micrograms/ 1 mL	IV bolus	May be diluted with N/S or G.	Give slowly, preferably over 10–15 minutes	**Acute events that may accompany administration:** Bradycardia, monitor heart rate and blood pressure. Rapid administration may produce transient hypertension and then hypotension. **pH:** 4–4.5 **Flush:** N/S **Sodium content:** Negligible	
	(C) IV infusion (unlicensed ICU practice)	Dilute in G (e.g. 600 micrograms in 30mL).			

Formulation	Method	Dilution	Rate	Comments	Compatibility
Co-amoxiclav					
Vial 600mg, containing amoxicillin 500mg and clavulanic acid 100mg and 1.2g containing amoxicillin 1g and clavulanic acid 200mg	IV bolus (preferred method). Use reconstituted injection within 20 minutes of preparation.	Reconstitute 600mg with 10mL and 1.2g with 20mL W.	3–4 minutes	**pH:** 8.8–9 **Flush:** N/S **Sodium content:** 1.6mmol/600mg, 2.7mmol/1.2g **Potassium content:** 0.5mmol/600mg, 1mmol/1.2g **Displacement:** 0.5mL/600mg, 0.9mL/1.2g Add 9.5mL W to 600mg vial to give a concentration of 600mg/10mL. Add 19.1mL W to 1.2g vial to give a concentration of 1.2g/20mL. **Other comments:** discard unused infusion after 4 hours. A transient pink coloration may appear during reconstitution. Reconstituted solutions are normally a pale-straw colour.	**Incompatible:** aminoglycosides
	(I) IV infusion	Reconstitute as above then dilute 600mg to 50mL and 1.2g with 100mL N/S.	30–40 minutes		

- For abbreviations used in the Table, see Section A, 2.4.
  e.g. (C) IV = continuous intravenous infusion; (I) IV = intermittent intravenous infusion.
- Prepare a fresh infusion every 24 hours unless otherwise specified.
- Presume suitability as single-use only unless otherwise specified.
- Always check with additional reference sources regarding compatibility information – see Section A, 2.2.

Formulation	Method	Dilution	Rate	Comments	Compatibility
Co-trimoxazole					
Ampoule 480mg/5mL, 960mg/10mL containing trimethoprim 1 part to sulfamethoxazole 5 parts	(I) IV infusion	Dilute each 480mg (5mL) to 125mL, 960mg (10mL) to 250mL, 1440mg (15mL) to 500mL, 1920mg (20mL) and 2400mg (25mL) to 500–1000mL with N/S, G or G/S.	Give over at least 60–90 minutes. Give over 2 hours if causing nausea	**Acute events that may accompany administration:** Nausea and vomiting. Thrombophlebitis at site of infusion. Localised pain and irritation during infusion. Extravasation may cause tissue damage; for management guidelines see Section A, 7. **pH:** 9–10.5 **Flush:** N/S **Sodium content:** 1.64mmol/480mg **Other comments:** More stable in G than N/S. Discard diluted infusion within 6 hours of preparation. Monitor all infusions carefully for cloudiness and precipitate formation. Do not refrigerate.	**Y-site compatible (but see Section A, 2.6):** aciclovir (both medicines in G), atracurium (both medicines in G), magnesium sulphate (both medicines in G), morphine (both medicines in G), pancuronium (both medicines in G). **Incompatible:** fluconazole, insulin (soluble), midazolam.
		Local practice on UCLH HIV and haematology wards: doses <40mL (3840mg) in 500mL G. Doses of 40mL (3840mg) or more in 1000mL N/S.	90 minutes to 2 hours		
	(I) IV infusion via syringe pump into a central line (unlicensed)	Undiluted (local practice).	90 minutes		

Formulation	Method	Dilution	Rate	Comments	Compatibility
Cyclizine					
Ampoule 50mg/1 mL	IV bolus	May be diluted 1:1 with W.	3–5 minutes	**Acute events that may accompany administration:** Hypotension and tachycardia, monitor blood pressure and heart rate. Pain at injection site. Extravasation may cause tissue damage; for management guidelines see Section A, 7. **pH:** 3.3–3.7 **Flush:** W or N/S **Sodium content:** Nil **Other comments:** More stable in W than N/S.	**Compatibility in S/C syringe pump:** with diamorphine see Section A 8 for details. **Incompatible:** all solutions of pH greater than 6.8; octreotide.
	(I) or (C) IV or S/C infusion (unlicensed)	May be diluted with W or N/S (local practice).			
	IM	Ready diluted.			

- For abbreviations used in the Table, see Section A, 2.4.
  e.g. (C) IV = continuous intravenous infusion; (I) IV = intermittent intravenous infusion.
- Prepare a fresh infusion every 24 hours unless otherwise specified.
- Presume suitability as single-use only unless otherwise specified.
- Always check with additional reference sources regarding compatibility information – see Section A, 2.2.

83

Formulation	Method	Dilution	Rate	Comments	Compatibility
Dalteparin					
Pre-filled syringe 2500 units/0.2 mL, 5000 units/ 0.2 mL, 7500 units/0.3 mL, 12500 units/ 0.5 mL, 15000 units/0.6 mL, 18000 units/ 0.72 mL. Graduated syringe: 10000 units/1 mL	S/C	Ready diluted.		**pH:** 5–7.5 **Flush:** N/S or G **Other comments:** IV administration is licensed only for the prevention of clotting in the extracorporeal circulation during haemodialysis or haemofiltration in patients with chronic renal insufficiency or acute renal failure. The S/C route is licensed for unstable angina, surgical thromboprophylaxis and treatment of VTE.	
Ampoule 100000 units/ 4 mL, 10000 units/1 mL	IV bolus	May be diluted with N/S or G.			
	(I) or (C) IV infusion.	May be diluted with N/S or G.			

Formulation	Method	Dilution	Rate	Comments	Compatibility
Dantrolene					
Vial 20mg	IV bolus	Reconstitute 20mg with 60mL W.	Give rapidly	**Acute events that may accompany administration:** Give centrally if possible because of high pH. If given peripherally care is needed to avoid extravasation as it may cause tissue damage; for management guidelines see Section A, 7. **pH:** 9.5 **Flush:** W **Sodium content:** 0.08 mmol/20mg vial **Other comments:** Discard 6 hours after reconstitution.	**Incompatible:** do not give with other medicines or infusion fluids including G and N/S.
	(I) IV infusion (used for prophylaxis of preoperative malignant hyperthermia)	As above, do not dilute further.	1 hour		

• For abbreviations used in the Table, see Section A, 2.4.
  e.g. (C) IV = continuous intravenous infusion; (I) IV = intermittent intravenous infusion.
• Prepare a fresh infusion every 24hours unless otherwise specified.
• Presume suitability as single-use only unless otherwise specified.
• Always check with additional reference sources regarding compatibility information – see Section A, 2.2.

Formulation	Method	Dilution	Rate	Comments	Compatibility
Desferrioxamine					
Vial 500mg	(I) or (C) IV infusion	Reconstitute each 500mg with 5mL W to give a 10% solution. This may be further diluted with N/S, G or G/S.	**Chronic iron overload:** 8–12 hours. Some patients may require administration over 24 hours. **Maintenance haemodialysis/ filtration:** infuse IV dose in 100mL N/S over the last 30–60 minutes of dialysis.	**Acute events that may accompany administration: Anaphylactoid** reactions, fever and muscle aches. IV bolus may lead to circulatory collapse. Concentrations of greater than 10% will increase the risk of local skin reactions if administered S/C. **pH:** 3.5–6.5 **Flush:** N/S **Displacement:** 0.4mL/500mg Add 4.6mL diluent to 500mg vial to give a concentration of 500mg in 5mL. **Other comments:** Discard infusion if cloudy. May also be added to CAPD bags.	Up to 10mg hydrocortisone sodium succinate may be added to 60mL Baxter elastomeric infusors and this should remain stable for 14 days. **Incompatible:** heparin
	(I) or (C) S/C infusion	As above.			
	IM	Reconstitute each 500mg with 5mL W. Can inject dose in two injections.			

Formulation	Method	Dilution	Rate	Comments	Compatibility
Desmopressin					
Ampoule 4 micrograms/ 1 mL, 15 micrograms/ 1 mL	(I) IV infusion	Dilute dose with 50 mL N/S.	20–30 minutes	**Acute events that may accompany administration:** Tachycardia and hypotension, monitor blood pressure continuously during infusions. Fluid overload likely, restrict fluid intake and check body weight regularly. **pH:** 4 **Flush:** N/S	
	IM or S/C	Ready diluted.			

- For abbreviations used in the Table, see Section A, 2.4.
  e.g. (C) IV = continuous intravenous infusion; (I) IV = intermittent intravenous infusion.
- Prepare a fresh infusion every 24 hours unless otherwise specified.
- Presume suitability as single-use only unless otherwise specified.
- Always check with additional reference sources regarding compatibility information – see Section A, 2.2.

87

Formulation	Method	Dilution	Rate	Comments	Compatibility
Dexamethasone					
All preparations come as dexamethasone sodium phosphate.

Mayne brand: dexamethasone phosphate 4mg/mL 1mL ampoule; 2mL vial; 5mL vial

Organon brand: dexamethasone 4mg/mL 1mL ampoule; 2mL vial | IV bolus | May be diluted with N/S or G. | Min. 3 minutes | **Acute events that may accompany administration:** Rapid administration may cause cardiovascular collapse. Serious anaphylactoid reactions, e.g. bronchospasm, have occurred. Perineal burning may be reduced by a longer administration period.
pH: 7–8.5
Flush: N/S
Sodium content: 0.021 mmol/1 mL
Other comments: The last dose should preferably be given before 6pm to avoid insomnia. | **Y-site compatible (but see Section A, 2.6):** aminophylline, fluconazole, heparin, granisetron, metoclopramide, morphine.
Compatibility in syringe pump for S/C administration: with diamorphine, see Section A, 8 for details.
Incompatible: octreotide, vancomycin. |
| | (I) IV infusion | Dilute in 100mL N/S or G. | 15 minutes | | |
| | S/C or IM | Dilution not required. | | | |

Formulation	Method	Dilution	Rate	Comments	Compatibility
Diamorphine					
Ampoule 5mg, 10mg, 30mg, 100mg, 500mg	IV bolus	Reconstitute 5mg, 10mg, 30mg and 100mg ampoules with 1 mL W. Reconstitute 500mg ampoule with 2mL W. May be diluted with G or N/S (preferably G).	3–5 minutes (local practice); 1mg/minute for treating myocardial infarction.	**Acute events that may accompany administration:** Severe respiratory depression, apnoea, hypotension, peripheral circulatory collapse, chest wall rigidity, cardiac arrest and anaphylactic shock. Monitor blood pressure, heart and respiratory rate. **pH:** 3.8–4.4 **Flush:** N/S or G **Sodium content:** Nil **Displacement:** Negligible **Other comments:** IV infusion is more stable in G than N/S.	**Compatibility in S/C syringe pump:** See Section A, 8 for details. **Incompatible:** alkaline agents
	(C) IV infusion via syringe pump	As above for reconstitution. Dilute with G or N/S (preferably G) to a convenient volume.			
	(C) S/C infusion via syringe pump	To reconstitute ampoule, see IV bolus above. Dilute with W if to be added to other compatible medicines. Dilute with N/S if not to be mixed with other medicines. Dilute to a convenient volume.			
	IM or S/C	As for IV			

- For abbreviations used in the Table, see Section A, 2.4.
  e.g. (C) IV = continuous intravenous infusion; (I) IV = intermittent intravenous infusion.
- Prepare a fresh infusion every 24hours unless otherwise specified.
- Presume suitability as single-use only unless otherwise specified.
- Always check with additional reference sources regarding compatibility information – see Section A, 2.2.

Formulation	Method	Dilution	Rate	Comments	Compatibility
Diazepam					
Ampoule 10mg/2mL	(C) IV infusion – not recommended. Use diazepam emulsion			**Acute events that may accompany administration:** Apnoea and hypotension, monitor respiratory rate and blood pressure. Circulatory and respiratory depression, monitor heart and respiratory rate. There is a higher incidence of vein irritation compared with diazepam emulsion. Extravasation may cause tissue damage; for management guidelines see Section A, 7. **pH:** 6.2–7.0 **Other comments:** Discard unused solution within 6 hours. Avoid contact with PVC administration sets. **Sodium content:** Nil	**Incompatible:** buprenorphine, doxapram, furosemide, flucloxacillin, glycopyrronium, heparin, ranitidine.
	IV bolus – not recommended. Use diazepam emulsion				
	IM – Only use when oral or IV dosing is not possible or advisable because absorption is variable	Ready diluted.			

Formulation	Method	Dilution	Rate	Comments	Compatibility
Diazepam emulsion					
Ampoule 10 mg/2 mL	IV bolus	Ready diluted.	5 mg/minute	**Acute events that may accompany administration:** Apnoea and hypotension, monitor respiratory rate and blood pressure. Circulatory and respiratory depression, monitor heart and respiratory rate. **pH:** 8 **Flush:** N/S **Other comments:** discard solution after 6 hours. Diazepam emulsion causes less local pain and thrombophlebitis compared with diazepam injection. Adsorption may occur to PVC infusion equipment. This occurs to a greater extent with diazepam injection. IV infusion best administered in specialist centres with ITU facilities. Not to be used if patient egg or soybean sensitive.	**Y-site compatible (but see Section A, 2.6):** N/S.
	(C) IV infusion via a syringe pump	Dilute with G or G 10% to achieve a concentration within the range 0.1– 0.4 mg/1 mL (i.e. 1–4 mL in 50 mL G).	Titrate rate to response Max: rate 125 micrograms/kg per hour		

- For abbreviations used in the Table, see Section A, 2.4.
  e.g. (C) IV = continuous intravenous infusion; (I) IV = intermittent intravenous infusion.
- Prepare a fresh infusion every 24 hours unless otherwise specified.
- Presume suitability as single-use only unless otherwise specified.
- Always check with additional reference sources regarding compatibility information – see Section A, 2.2.

Formulation	Method	Dilution	Rate	Comments	Compatibility
Diazoxide					
Ampoule 300 mg/20 mL	IV bolus – emergency use only (max. dose 150 mg)	Do not dilute.	Give rapidly (<30 seconds)	**Acute events that may accompany administration:** Hyperglycaemia, monitor blood glucose levels regularly. Reflex tachycardia in the first few minutes after injection. Pain or a feeling of warmth along injected vein. Extravasation may cause tissue damage; for management guidelines see Section A, 7. **pH:** 11.6 **Flush:** N/S **Sodium content:** 1.5 mmol/300 mg **Other comments:** Dose may be repeated after 5–15 minutes if necessary. Slow administration reduces the antihypertensive response. Note: the BNF indicates that this is a product less suitable for prescribing.	

Formulation	Method	Dilution	Rate	Comments	Compatibility
Diclofenac					
Ampoule 75mg/3mL	(I) IV infusion	Buffer 100–500mL N/S or G with sodium bicarbonate solution (0.5mL 8.4% or 1mL 4.2%). Add one ampoule of diclofenac to the infusion bag.	25–50mg over 15–60 minutes. 75mg over 30–120 minutes	**Acute events that may accompany administration:** IM injection may cause site reactions, abscesses and local necrosis. Hypersensitivity reactions to excipients. **pH:** 7.8–9 **Flush:** N/S or G **Sodium content:** Negligible **Other comments:** Maximum duration of parenteral treatment is 2 consecutive days. Administer IM injection by deep intragluteal injection into the upper quadrant. If necessary use alternate buttock for second injection.	Do not infuse with other medicines.
	(C) IV infusion	As above.	Approximately 5mg/hour		
	IM See 'Other comments'	Ready diluted.			

- For abbreviations used in the Table, see Section A, 2.4.
  e.g. (C) IV = continuous intravenous infusion; (I) IV = intermittent intravenous infusion.
- Prepare a fresh infusion every 24 hours unless otherwise specified.
- Presume suitability as single-use only unless otherwise specified.
- Always check with additional reference sources regarding compatibility information – see Section A, 2.2.

93

Formulation	Method	Dilution	Rate	Comments	Compatibility
Dicobalt edetate					
Ampoule 300 mg/20 mL	IV bolus	Ready diluted.	Max. rate 300 mg/minute If patient's condition is less serious give dose over 5 minutes	**Acute events that may accompany administration:** Can cause hypotension and tachycardia. **pH:** 4–7.5 **Flush:** G **Sodium content:** Nil **Other comments:** Each dose may be followed immediately with 50 mL G 50%. In the absence of cyanide, dicobalt edetate is itself toxic.	**Y-site compatible (but see Section A, 2.6):** G, W.

Formulation	Method	Dilution	Rate	Comments	Compatibility
Digoxin					
Ampoule 500 micrograms/ 2 mL, 100 micrograms/ 1 mL (paediatric)	(I) IV infusion via syringe or volumetric infusion pump (preferred method)	Dilute 1 part digoxin with at least 4 parts N/S, G or G/S. Volume of final solution for adults is usually 50–100 mL (max. 500 mL).	Usually 2 or more hours. Min. time: 10– 20 minutes	**Acute events that may accompany administration:** Arrhythmias, monitor heart rate and **ECG** recommended. Rapid administration may cause nausea and risk of arrhythmias and/or reduced coronary flow. Rapid injection may cause vasoconstriction and transient hypertension; monitor blood pressure. **pH:** 6.7–7.3 **Flush:** N/S **Other comments:** The IM route is rarely justified because it causes severe local irritation and results in unreliable absorption.	**Y-site compatible (but see Section A, 2.6):** ciprofloxacin, flucloxacillin, furosemide, heparin, insulin (soluble), lidocaine, morphine, potassium chloride, verapamil. **Incompatible:** dobutamine, doxapram, foscarnet.
	IV bolus	Dilute 1 part digoxin with at least 4 parts N/S, G or G/S. Fluid restriction: can give undiluted, but if diluting then do so as above.	Min. time: 10 minutes		
	IM See 'Other comments'	Ready diluted.			

- For abbreviations used in the Table, see Section A, 2.4.
  e.g. (C) IV = continuous intravenous infusion; (I) IV = intermittent intravenous infusion.
- Prepare a fresh infusion every 24 hours unless otherwise specified.
- Presume suitability as single-use only unless otherwise specified.
- Always check with additional reference sources regarding compatibility information – see Section A, 2.2.

Formulation	Method	Dilution	Rate	Comments	Compatibility
Digoxin-specific antibody fragments (Digibind)					
Vial 38mg	(I) IV infusion	Reconstitute vial with 4mL W. May be diluted with N/S to a suitable volume. Administer through 0.2 μm sterile disposable filter.	30 minutes	**Acute events that may accompany administration:** Continuous ECG monitoring for 24 hours after administration of Digibind. Significant hypokalaemia can occur; monitor potassium levels. Allergic reactions, rash, shaking and chills without fever can occur. **pH:** 6–8 **Flush:** N/S **Sodium content:** 0.47mmol/vial **Other comments:** The reconstituted vial should be stored in the refrigerator and used within 4 hours.	Do not infuse with other medicines.
	IV bolus (use if cardiac arrest seems imminent)	Reconstitute vial with 4mL of W.	3–5 minutes		

Formulation	Method	Dilution	Rate	Comments	Compatibility
Disopyramide					
Ampoule 50mg/5mL	IV bolus (max. dose 150mg)	Ready diluted.	Min. time: 5 minutes. Max. rate 30mg/minute	**Acute events that may accompany administration:** If given too quickly profuse sweating and cardiovascular depression may occur. Monitor blood pressure and **ECG.** Preferred route is peripheral because central administration may cause hypotension and cardiac arrest. **pH:** 4.5 **Flush:** N/S **Other comments:** Maximum dose 300mg in first hour and 800mg in 24 hours (including loading dose).	Do not infuse with other medicines.
	(C) IV infusion following loading dose as IV bolus. Use syringe or volumetric infusion pump	Dilute with N/S, G, H or Ringer's.	20–30mg/hour or 0.4mg/kg per hour		

- For abbreviations used in the Table, see Section A, 2.4.
  e.g. (C) IV = continuous intravenous infusion; (I) IV = intermittent intravenous infusion.
- Prepare a fresh infusion every 24 hours unless otherwise specified.
- Presume suitability as single-use only unless otherwise specified.
- Always check with additional reference sources regarding compatibility information – see Section A, 2.2.

97

Formulation	Method	Dilution	Rate	Comments	Compatibility
Dobutamine					
Ampoule 250mg/20mL	(C) IV infusion via syringe pump	Dilute to 0.5–1mg/mL (usual max. 5mg/1mL) with N/S or G. Concentrations of up to 10mg/1mL or even undiluted have been used via a central line (unlicensed local practice). Strengths >5mg/mL should preferably be given centrally.		**Acute events that may accompany administration:** Heart rate, rhythm and arterial blood pressure should be closely monitored. The use of dobutamine should be restricted to areas where full haemodynamic monitoring is available. Extravasation may cause tissue damage; for management guidelines see Section A, 7. **pH:** 2.5–5.5 **Do not flush:** Replace giving set **Sodium content:** Negligible **Other comments:** Solution may turn pink. This is due to a slight oxidation of the medicine and is harmless. Prepared solutions stable for 24 hours at room temperature.	**Y-site compatible (but see Section A, 2.6):** adrenaline (epinephrine), amiodarone, atropine, bretylium, calcium chloride, calcium gluconate, ciprofloxacin, diazepam, dopamine, glyceryl trinitrate, hydralazine, isoprenaline, lidocaine, magnesium sulphate, noradrenaline (norepinephrine) (local practice), pancuronium, phenylephrine, potassium chloride, procainamide (in N/S). **Incompatible:** aciclovir, alteplase, aminophylline, amphotericin, bumetanide, digoxin, furosemide, sodium bicarbonate and other strong alkaline agents.

Formulation	Method	Dilution	Rate	Comments	Compatibility
Dopamine					
Ampoule 200 mg/5 mL, Infusion 400 mg/250 mL	(C) IV infusion via a volumetric infusion or syringe pump. See 'Other comments'	Dilute with N/S, G or H to a suggested maximum concentration of 1.6 mg/1 mL (800 mg in 500 mL). Concentrations up to 8 mg/1 mL have been used (unlicensed). A dilution of 200 mg in 50 mL is used routinely on the ICUs (local practice). See 'Other comments' for choice of route of administration.		**Acute events that may accompany administration:** When administered peripherally, extravasation can produce local vasoconstriction, leading to severe tissue hypoxia and ischaemia; for general treatment guidelines see Section A, 7. If extravasation occurs irrigate affected area with 5–10 mg phentolamine in 10–15 mL N/S. Observe infusion site carefully. **ECG** monitoring is usually required but is not essential for low dose (1–3 micrograms/kg per minute) infusions. **pH:** 2.5–5.5 **Do not flush:** Replace giving set **Sodium content:** 0.52 mmol/200 mg **Other comments:** Administration via a central line is advisable and for concentrations >2 mg/1 mL is essential. If given peripherally use a dilute solution (1.6 mg/1 mL or less) and administer via a large vein. Solution is stable for 24 hours at room temperature. Protect from light; do not use if discoloured. **Paediatric information:** Use a central venous line for concentrations >2 mg/1 mL and doses over 10 micrograms/kg per minute.	**Y-site compatible (but see Section A, 2.6):** adrenaline (epinephrine), aminophylline, amiodarone, atracurium, bretylium, chloramphenicol, ciprofloxacin, dobutamine, doxapram, glyceryl trinitrate, heparin, insulin (soluble), labetalol, lidocaine, mannitol, noradrenaline (norepinephrine), potassium chloride, sodium nitroprusside. **Incompatible:** aciclovir, alteplase, amphotericin, sodium bicarbonate, other alkaline agents.

- For abbreviations used in the Table, see Section A, 2.4.
  e.g. (C) IV = continuous intravenous infusion; (I) IV = intermittent intravenous infusion.
- Prepare a fresh infusion every 24 hours unless otherwise specified.
- Presume suitability as single-use only unless otherwise specified.
- Always check with additional reference sources regarding compatibility information – see Section A, 2.2.

Formulation	Method	Dilution	Rate	Comments	Compatibility
Doxapram					
Ampoule 100 mg/5 mL, infusion bottle 1 g in 500 mL G	(C) IV infusion via volumetric infusion pump	Provided as ready diluted solution of 1 g in 500 mL G.	Rate control recommended. **Adults:** titrate dose. Usual max. rate 4 mg/minute	**Acute events that may accompany administration:** Moderate increase in blood pressure and slight increase in heart rate. Extravasation may cause tissue damage; for management guidelines see Section A, 7. **pH:** 3–5 **Flush:** N/S or G **Other comments:** Single bolus injections should not exceed 1.5 mg/kg.	**Y-site compatible (but see Section A, 2.6):** adrenaline (epinephrine), bumetanide, dopamine, potassium chloride, terbutaline. **Incompatible:** alkaline agents, e.g. aminophylline, cefuroxime, diazepam, digoxin, furosemide, ketamine, sodium bicarbonate.
	IV bolus	May be diluted with N/S, G or G 10%.	Min. 30 seconds		

Formulation	Method	Dilution	Rate	Comments	Compatibility
Drotrecogin alfa					
Vial 5 mg, 20 mg	(C) IV infusion	Reconstitute vials with W as below: **5 mg with 2.5 mL or 20 mg with 10 mL,** resulting in a 2 mg/mL solution. Avoid inverting or shaking the vial. Dilute this solution with N/S to a final concentration between 100 micrograms/mL and 200 micrograms/mL, e.g. patient weight 40–66 kg: 10 mg in 100 mL (100 micrograms/mL) or patient weight 67–135 kg: 20 mg in 100 mL (200 micrograms/mL).	24 micrograms/kg per hour for 96 hours	**Acute events that may accompany administration:** Increased risk of bleeding; headache, ecchymosis and pain. **pH:** 5.6–6.4 **Flush:** N/S **Sodium content:** 5 mg–0.7 mmol, 20 mg–2.6 mmol **Displacement:** Not known **Other comments:** Store at 2–8°C and protect from light. After reconstitution vials maybe stored for up to 3 hours at room temperature. Diluted solutions are stable for up to 14 hours at room temperature.	**Y-site compatible (but see Section A, 2.3):** glyceryl trinitrate, vasopressin, potassium chloride. **Incompatible:** adrenaline (epinephrine), albumin, amiodarone, ciclosporin, dobutamine, dopamine, furosemide, gentamicin, heparin, insulin (soluble), magnesium sulphate, midazolam, sodium nitroprusside, noradrenaline (norepinephrine), piperacillin/ tazobactam, vancomycin.

- For abbreviations used in the Table, see Section A, 2.4.
  e.g. (C) IV = continuous intravenous infusion; (I) IV = intermittent intravenous infusion.
- Prepare a fresh infusion every 24 hours unless otherwise specified.
- Presume suitability as single-use only unless otherwise specified.
- Always check with additional reference sources regarding compatibility information – see Section A, 2.2.

101

Formulation	Method	Dilution	Rate	Comments	Compatibility
Enoximone					
Ampoule 100 mg/20 mL	(C) IV infusion (preferred method)	Dilute with an equal volume of N/S, e.g. 100 mg/20 mL with 20 mL N/S to make 100 mg/40 mL.	See manufacturer's literature	**Acute events that may accompany administration:** Arrhythmias, hypotension, headache, diarrhoea, chills, oliguria, pain. **pH:** 12 (11.0 once diluted) **Flush:** N/S **Sodium content:** 0.6 mmol/100 mg **Displacement:** None. **Other comments:** Do NOT use more dilute solutions or use G as the diluent as precipitation may occur. Do NOT use glass syringes/ containers as crystals can form within 1 hour.	**Incompatible:** G insulin (soluble), furosemide.
	(I) IV infusion	As above.	See manufacturer's literature		

Formulation	Method	Dilution	Rate	Comments	Compatibility
Ephedrine					
Ampoule 30mg/1mL	IV bolus	Dilute to 3mg in 1mL with N/S, G or G/S.	3–5 minutes	**Acute events that may accompany administration:** Hypo-/hypertension, brady-/tachycardia. Monitor blood pressure and heart rate. CNS disturbances. **pH:** 4.5–7 **Flush:** N/S	**Compatible:** metaraminol, propofol. **Incompatible:** hydrocortisone sodium succinate, phenobarbital, thiopental.
	IM (unlicensed)	Ready diluted.			

- For abbreviations used in the Table, see Section A, 2.4.
  e.g. (C) IV = continuous intravenous infusion; (I) IV = intermittent intravenous infusion.
- Prepare a fresh infusion every 24 hours unless otherwise specified.
- Presume suitability as single-use only unless otherwise specified.
- Always check with additional reference sources regarding compatibility information – see Section A, 2.2.

103

Formulation	Method	Dilution	Rate	Comments	Compatibility
Epoprostenol (prostacyclin)					
Vial 500000 nanograms	(C) IV infusion via syringe or volumetric. infusion pump	Reconstitute using the 50mL diluent provided to prepare a concentrate containing 10000 nanograms/ 1mL. Prime the filter with concentrate before measuring the required dose. Dilute each 1 part concentrate (using filter provided) with a maximum of 6 parts N/S, e.g. 50mL of concentrate with a maximum of 300mL N/S. Prime giving set fully before commencing infusion.	See package insert or local policy on epoprostenol in the treatment of peripheral-vascular disease	**Acute events that may accompany administration:** Tachycardia, bradycardia, hypotension, monitor blood pressure and heart rate. A bright redness over the line of vein; exclude infection and treat with an NSAID. Headache, facial flushing, nausea, vomiting, abdominal cramps and jaw pain. Extravasation may cause tissue damage; for management guidelines see Section A, 7. **pH:** (of diluent) 10.5 **Do not flush:** Replace giving set after each administration **Sodium content:** 2.5mmol/reconstituted vial **Displacement:** Negligible **Other comments:** Discard any unused infusion after 12 hours. Some centres extend to 24 hours with no discernible loss of efficacy – unlicensed. Do not stop infusion for more than a few minutes. **Neonatal information:** Epoprostenol has an antiplatelet effect so heparin should not be added to the infusion bag.	Do not infuse with other medicines including G and G/S.

104

Formulation	Method	Dilution	Rate	Comments	Compatibility
		May also be administered into the blood supplying the dialyser. Fluid restricted: the concentrate may be administered undiluted (10 micrograms/mL) (unlicensed).			

- For abbreviations used in the Table, see Section A, 2.4.
  e.g. (C) IV = continuous intravenous infusion; (I) IV = intermittent intravenous infusion.
- Prepare a fresh infusion every 24 hours unless otherwise specified.
- Presume suitability as single-use only unless otherwise specified.
- Always check with additional reference sources regarding compatibility information – see Section A, 2.2.

Formulation	Method	Dilution	Rate	Comments	Compatibility
Eptifibatide					
Vial 75mg/100mL for infusion, 20mg/10mL for bolus	IV bolus (immediately followed by infusion)	Withdraw dose required from the 2mg/1mL (20mg/10mL) vial for injection and inject undiluted.	1 minute	**Acute events that may accompany administration: Bleeding,** particularly when cardiac catheterisation is via femoral artery access site; remove sheath when coagulation has returned to normal. Thrombocytopenia: monitor platelet count before treatment and 4–6 hours after bolus dose, and once daily if infusion is continued. Seek haematologist's advice if platelet count decreases. **pH:** 5–5.5 **Flush:** N/S **Displacement:** N/A **Sodium content:** Nil **Other comments:** The infusion vial may be used for up to 96 hours; once opened, discard any unused product after completion of infusion.	**Incompatible:** furosemide
	(C) IV infusion (immediately following bolus)	75mg/100mL vial for infusion – ready diluted.	See manufacturer's literature		

106

Formulation	Method	Dilution	Rate	Comments	Compatibility
Ergometrine					
500 micrograms/ 1 mL	IV bolus (but IM route preferred)	Dilute with 5 mL N/S.	Min. 1 minute.	**Acute events that may accompany administration:** Nausea and vomiting. Hypertension, bradycardia, palpitations, headache, dizziness and tinnitus may all occur if administered too quickly or undiluted. Extravasation may cause tissue damage; for management guidelines see Section A, 7. **pH:** 2.7–3.5 **Flush:** N/S	
	IM (preferred route)	Ready diluted.			

- For abbreviations used in the Table, see Section A, 2.4.
  e.g. (C) IV = continuous intravenous infusion; (I) IV = intermittent intravenous infusion.
- Prepare a fresh infusion every 24 hours unless otherwise specified.
- Presume suitability as single-use only unless otherwise specified.
- Always check with additional reference sources regarding compatibility information – see Section A, 2.2.

107

Formulation	Method	Dilution	Rate	Comments	Compatibility
Erythromycin (as lactobionate)					
Vial 1 g	(I) IV infusion	Reconstitute each 1 g with 20 mL W to produce 50 mg/1 mL, then further dilute to a maximum concentration of 5 mg/1 mL with N/S (e.g. 500 mg in 100 mL). G or G/S may be used instead of N/S, but add 5 mL sodium bicarbonate 8.4%/L of diluent as a buffer.	20–60 minutes. Patients at risk of arrhythmias (especially those associated with QT prolongation); should be given no more than 10 mg/minute	**Acute events that may accompany administration:** IV infusion may cause thrombophlebitis; check injection site. Arrhythmias may occur when administered as described for fluid-restricted patients; **ECG** monitoring is required. **pH:** 6.5–7.5 (reconstituted vial) **Flush:** N/S **Sodium content:** Nil **Displacement:** Is allowed for Add 20 mL W to 1 g vial to give a concentration of 1 g in 20 mL (50 mg in 1 mL). **Other comments:** Reconstituted solutions (50 mg/mL) may be kept at 2–8°C for 24 hours. Prepare a fresh infusion every 8 hours.	**Y-site compatible (but see Section A, 2.6):** aciclovir, aminophylline, magnesium sulphate. **Incompatible:** fluconazole, heparin, gentamicin and all other solutions of pH <5.5.

Formulation	Method	Dilution	Rate	Comments	Compatibility
	(C) IV infusion	Reconstitute as above then dilute as above to a max. concentration of 1 mg/1 mL.			
	(I) IV infusion via a central line for fluid-restricted patients (unlicensed)	Reconstitute each 1 g with 20 mL W to produce 50 mg/1 mL then dilute 1 g to 100 mL with N/S.	Min. 60 minutes.		

- For abbreviations used in the Table, see Section A, 2.4.
  e.g. (C) IV = continuous intravenous infusion; (I) IV = intermittent intravenous infusion.
- Prepare a fresh infusion every 24 hours unless otherwise specified.
- Presume suitability as single-use only unless otherwise specified.
- Always check with additional reference sources regarding compatibility information – see Section A, 2.2.

Formulation	Method	Dilution	Rate	Comments	Compatibility
Esmolol hydrochloride					
100 mg/10 mL vial, 2500 mg/ 250 mL bag, 2500 mg/10 mL ampoule	(C) IV infusion	100 mg/10 mL vial and 2500 mg/250 mL bag are pre-diluted, ready to use. 2500 mg/10 mL must be diluted with N/S or G to a 10 mg/mL solution. Diluted solution is stable for 24 hours at room temperature.	Loading dose: refer to SPC for specific instructions. Usual maintenance dose: 50–200 micrograms/kg per minute, titrate to response. Refer to SPC for specific instructions.	**Acute events that may accompany administration:** Hypotension, bradycardia, heart block, depressed myocardial contractility, peripheral constriction. Monitor heart rate and blood pressure frequently; bronchospasm. Concentrations >10 mg/mL into small veins or through butterfly catheter are associated with increased venous irritation and thrombophlebitis – AVOID. **pH:** Ready to use: 4.5–5.5; concentrate: 3.5–5.5 **Flush:** N/S or G **Sodium content:** Approximately 0.02 mmol/mL in 100 mg/10 mL injection; 0.12 mmol/mL in 2500 mg/250 mL premix injection; 0.12 mmol/mL in 2500 mg/10 mL concentrate. **Displacement:** N/A **Other comments:** Pharmacological adverse effects should resolve within 30 minutes of reducing dose or discontinuation.	**Y-site compatible (but see Section A, 2.3):** noradrenaline (norepinephrine) when reconstituted in G. **Incompatible:** sodium bicarbonate, thiopental, diazepam.
Etomidate					
Ampoule 20 mg/10 mL	IV bolus into large vein	May be diluted with N/S or G.	Min. 2 minutes.	**Acute events that may accompany administration:** There is a high incidence of muscle movement and pain on injection. Pain is reduced if a large vein is used. Diazepam or an opioid analgesic will reduce muscle movement. Hypotension can occur if given too quickly. **pH:** 4–7 **Flush:** N/S or G **Other comments:** Each ampoule contains 35% propylene glycol.	**Incompatible:** H, pancuronium, vecuronium.

Formulation	Method	Dilution	Rate	Comments	Compatibility
Fentanyl					
Ampoule 100 micrograms/1mL, 500 micrograms/10mL	IV bolus	May be diluted with N/S, G, G/S or H.	1–2 minutes	**Acute events that may accompany administration:** Muscular rigidity may occur with rapid injection. Severe respiratory depression, apnoea, peripheral circulatory collapse, chest wall rigidity, cardiac arrest and anaphylactic shock. Bradycardia and transient hypotension may occur, especially in hypovolaemic patients. Monitor blood pressure, heart and respiratory rate. Extravasation may cause tissue damage; for management guidelines see Section A, 7. **pH:** 4–7.5 **Flush:** N/S **Sodium content:** 0.3mmol/1mL	**Y-site compatible (but see Section A, 2.6):** atracurium, heparin, midazolam, mivacurium, pancuronium, potassium chloride, propofol, sodium bicarbonate. **Incompatible:** alkaline agents including thiopental.
	IM	Ready diluted.			

- For abbreviations used in the Table, see Section A, 2.4.
  e.g. (C) IV = continuous intravenous infusion; (I) IV = intermittent intravenous infusion.
- Prepare a fresh infusion every 24hours unless otherwise specified.
- Presume suitability as single-use only unless otherwise specified.
- Always check with additional reference sources regarding compatibility information – see Section A, 2.2.

Formulation	Method	Dilution	Rate	Comments	Compatibility
Filgrastim					
Vial 300 micrograms/ 1 mL (30 million units), 0.5 mL prefilled syringes (600 micrograms/ 1 mL, 960 micrograms/ 1 mL)	S/C	Ready diluted.		**Acute events that may accompany administration:** Pain on injection and erythema are more likely if administered rapidly intravenously. **pH:** 4 **Flush:** G **Sodium content:** Negligible **Other comments:** Filgrastim may be adsorbed on to glass and plastic, so do not dilute to a concentration of <2 micrograms/1 mL. Only clear solutions without particles should be used. Shaking of the injection should be avoided as frothing may occur. If this occurs leave vial to stand.	**Incompatible:** N/S
	(I) IV infusion	Preferred method of infusion: dilute with G to a minimum concentration of 15 micrograms/ 1 mL, i.e. dilute 300 micrograms filgrastim to 20mL G and give over 30 minutes. Local practice is preferentially to use the S/C route.	30 minutes		

Formulation	Method	Dilution	Rate	Comments	Compatibility
		If lower concentrations of 2–15 micrograms/1 mL are required, then human serum albumin solution should be added to the G to produce a final albumin concentration of 2 mg/mL before the filgrastim is added. A 4.5% solution of albumin contains 45 mg/1 mL.			

- For abbreviations used in the Table, see Section A, 2.4.

e.g. (C) IV = continuous intravenous infusion; (I) IV = intermittent intravenous infusion.

- Prepare a fresh infusion every 24 hours unless otherwise specified.
- Presume suitability as single-use only unless otherwise specified.
- Always check with additional reference sources regarding compatibility information – see Section A, 2.2.

Formulation	Method	Dilution	Rate	Comments	Compatibility
Flecainide					
Ampoule 150 mg/15 mL	IV bolus	May be diluted with G.	Min. 10 minutes.	**Acute events that may accompany administration:** Arrhythmias, monitor **ECG** continuously, if bolus doses are given. **pH:** 6–6.5 **Flush:** G **Other comments:** Do not use infusion as route of administration for longer than 24 hours.	**Y-site compatible (but see Section A, 2.6):** bretylium, digoxin, H, isosorbide dinitrate, streptokinase. **Incompatible:** alkaline agents and those containing chloride, phosphate or sulphate ions.
	(I) IV infusion. Preferred method for patients with cardiac failure or ventricular tachycardia	May be diluted with G.	Min. 30 minutes for patients with cardiac failure or ventricular tachycardia.		
	(C) IV infusion via volumetric infusion pump	See package insert. Dilute with G. If the diluent is N/S, use at least 500 mL to prevent precipitation.			

Formulation	Method	Dilution	Rate	Comments	Compatibility
Flucloxacillin					
Vial 250 mg, 500 mg	IV bolus (preferred method)	Reconstitute 250–500 mg with 5–10 mL and 1 g with 15–20 mL W. May be diluted with N/S, G or G/S.	3–5 minutes.	**Acute events that may accompany administration:** Anaphylaxis. **pH:** 5–7 (reconstituted) **Flush:** N/S **Sodium content:** 0.57 mmol/250 mg **Displacement:** 0.2 mL/250 mg Add 4.8 mL of diluent to 250 mg vial to give a concentration of 250 mg in 5 mL (50 mg in 1 mL).	**Y-site compatible (but see Section A, 2.6):** aminophylline, diamorphine, digoxin, heparin, potassium chloride, ranitidine. **Incompatible:** aminoglycosides, amiodarone, benzylpenicillin, ciprofloxacin, diazepam, morphine.
	(I) IV infusion	Reconstitute as above then dilute with N/S, G or G/S to 100 mL.	30–60 minutes.		
	IM	Reconstitute 250 mg with 1.5 mL and 500 mg with 2 mL W.			

- For abbreviations used in the Table, see Section A, 2.4.
  e.g. (C) IV = continuous intravenous infusion; (I) IV = intermittent intravenous infusion.
- Prepare a fresh infusion every 24 hours unless otherwise specified.
- Presume suitability as single-use only unless otherwise specified.
- Always check with additional reference sources regarding compatibility information – see Section A, 2.2.

Formulation	Method	Dilution	Rate	Comments	Compatibility
Fluconazole					
Vial 50mg/25mL, 200mg/100mL	(I) IV infusion	Ready diluted.	10–20mg/minute	**pH:** 4–8 **Flush:** N/S **Sodium content:** 15mmol/200mg (100mL bottle) No additions should be made to the fluconazole infusion.	**Y-site compatible (but see Section A, 2.6):** aciclovir, dexamethasone, folinic acid, foscarnet, ganciclovir, heparin, N/S, metronidazole, potassium chloride in G, vancomycin. **Incompatible:** amphotericin, calcium gluconate, ceftazidime, cefuroxime, erythromycin, furosemide, imipenem.
Flucytosine					
Infusion bottle 2.5g/250mL	(I) IV infusion	Ready diluted. Administer via a giving set incorporating a 15 µm filter.	20–40 minutes	**pH:** 7.4 **Flush:** N/S or G **Sodium content:** 34.5mmol/250mL **Other comments:** Must be stored between 18 and 25°C, otherwise precipitation of flucytosine may occur. Contact pharmacy if precipitation is visible. Prolonged storage above 25°C could lead to decomposition of flucytosine to 5-fluorouracil.	**Y-site compatible (but see Section A, 2.6):** N/S, G, or G/S **Incompatible:** do not infuse with other medicines.

Formulation	Method	Dilution	Rate	Comments	Compatibility
Flumazenil					
Ampoule 500 micrograms/ 5 mL	IV bolus	May be diluted with N/S or G.	Min. 15 seconds	**Acute events that may accompany administration:** Excessive and/or rapidly injected doses may induce benzodiazepine withdrawal symptoms. Transient increases in blood pressure, flushing and rarely seizures especially in patients with epilepsy. **pH:** 4 **Flush:** N/S **Other comments:** IV infusion may be useful if drowsiness recurs after IV bolus. Infusions should be used within 3 hours of preparation.	Do not infuse with other medicines.
	(I) IV infusion via volumetric infusion pump	As above.	100–400 micrograms/hour		

- For abbreviations used in the Table, see Section A, 2.4.
  e.g. (C) IV = continuous intravenous infusion; (I) IV = intermittent intravenous infusion.
- Prepare a fresh infusion every 24 hours unless otherwise specified.
- Presume suitability as single-use only unless otherwise specified.
- Always check with additional reference sources regarding compatibility information – see Section A, 2.2.

117

Formulation	Method	Dilution	Rate	Comments	Compatibility
Folic acid (unlicensed)					
Ampoule 15 mg/1 mL	IV bolus	May be diluted with a small volume of N/S, e.g. 10 mL.	3–5 minutes	**Acute events that may accompany administration:** Extravasation may cause tissue damage; for management guidelines, see Section A, 7. **pH:** 8–11 **Flush:** N/S	**Incompatible:** will precipitate at pH below 4.5–5.
	IM	Ready diluted.			

Formulation	Method	Dilution	Rate	Comments	Compatibility
Folinic acid (calcium folinate)					
Vial 15mg, 30mg, 350mg/35mL	IV bolus or (I) IV infusion	Reconstitute 15mg and 30mg vial with 3mL W. For IV infusion dilute with a suitable volume of N/S or G.	Max. rate 160mg/minute (350mg over at least 3–5 minutes).	**Acute events that may accompany administration:** Hypotension, vasomotor collapse, nausea, vomiting, hot flushes and sweating may occur if administered too rapidly because of the calcium content. **pH:** 6.5–8.6 **Flush:** N/S **Sodium content:** 0.2mmol/15mg, 0.4mmol/30mg, 4.6mmol/350mg vial. **Displacement:** 15mg and 30mg vial negligible **Other comments:** Folinic acid 350mg contains 0.7mmol calcium therefore administer slowly. Reconstituted solutions are intended for immediate administration but stable for 24 hours at 2–8°C.	**Y-site compatible (but see Section A, 2.6):** cisplatin, fluorouracil, fluconazole, piperacillin/tazobactam. **Incompatible:** trimetrexate, foscarnet.
	IM	Reconstitute 15mg and 30mg vial with 3mL W.			

- For abbreviations used in the Table, see Section A, 2.4.
  e.g. (C) IV = continuous intravenous infusion; (I) IV = intermittent intravenous infusion.
- Prepare a fresh infusion every 24 hours unless otherwise specified.
- Presume suitability as single-use only unless otherwise specified.
- Always check with additional reference sources regarding compatibility information – see Section A, 2.2.

Formulation	Method	Dilution	Rate	Comments	Compatibility
Foscarnet sodium					
Infusion bottle 24mg/1mL, 6g in 250mL, 12g in 500mL	(1) IV infusion via volumetric infusion pump	If given peripherally, dilute with N/S or G to at least 12mg/1mL. Local practice is to achieve this dilution by piggybacking 1L of N/S with the dose of foscarnet. If given centrally, can be administered undiluted but additional fluids should be given to reduce the risk of nephrotoxicity.	2 hours (local practice).	**Acute events that may accompany administration:** Pins and needles (paraesthesiae) due to transient hypocalcaemia. Peripheral administration may lead to local irritation and thrombophlebitis. **pH:** 7.4 (undiluted) **Flush:** N/S or G **Sodium content:** 15.6mmol/1g **Other comments:** If contact occurs it may cause local burning sensation; wash skin with water.	**Y-site compatible (but see Section A, 2.6):** cefuroxime, clindamycin, fluconazole, gentamicin, hydrocortisone sodium succinate, metronidazole. **Incompatible:** aciclovir, amphotericin, digoxin, ganciclovir, pentamidine. Any calcium-containing solutions.

120

Formulation	Method	Dilution	Rate	Comments	Compatibility
Furosemide					
Ampoule 20mg/2mL, 50mg/5mL, 250mg/25mL	IV bolus	May be diluted with N/S.	**Adults:** max. rate 4mg/minute.	**Acute events that may accompany administration:** Rapid administration may result in hearing disorders such as tinnitus and deafness. Extravasation may cause tissue damage; for management guidelines, see Section A, 7. **pH:** 8–9.5 **Flush:** N/S **Sodium content:** 0.3mmol for 20mg/2mL, 0.7mmol for 50mg/5mL, 4mmol for 250mg/25mL.	**Y-site compatible (but see Section A, 2.6):** aminophylline, atropine, bumetanide, digoxin, glyceryl trinitrate, heparin, hydrocortisone sodium succinate, insulin (soluble), lidocaine, magnesium sulphate, potassium chloride, ranitidine. **Incompatible:** amiodarone, amphotericin, bleomycin, ciprofloxacin, diazepam, dobutamine, doxapram, fluconazole, gentamicin, G, isoprenaline, metoclopramide, morphine, netilmicin, noradrenaline (norepinephrine), pethidine, vecuronium.
	(C) IV or (I) IV infusion via a syringe or volumetric infusion pump	Dilute with N/S or H to a convenient volume (or may be given undiluted).			

- For abbreviations used in the Table, see Section A, 2.4.
- e.g. (C) IV = continuous intravenous infusion; (I) IV = intermittent intravenous infusion.
- Prepare a fresh infusion every 24 hours unless otherwise specified.
- Presume suitability as single-use only unless otherwise specified.
- Always check with additional reference sources regarding compatibility information – see Section A, 2.2.

121

Formulation	Method	Dilution	Rate	Comments	Compatibility
Fusidic acid					
	See Sodium fusidate				
Ganciclovir					
Vial 500 mg	(I) IV infusion either centrally or via a large peripheral vein with good blood flow, preferably using a plastic cannula.	**Handle as for cytotoxic medicines** Reconstitute each 500 mg with 10 mL W. Dilute to a concentration not exceeding 10 mg/1 mL with N/S or G.	Min. 60 minutes.	**Acute events that may accompany administration:** Pain on infusion, can cause thrombophlebitis. Extravasation may cause tissue damage; for management guidelines, see Section A, 7. **pH:** 10–11 (reconstituted vial) **Flush:** N/S or G **Sodium content:** 2 mmol/500 mg **Displacement:** 0.29 mL/500 mg. Add 9.7 mL diluent to 500 mg vial to give a concentration of 500 mg/10 mL. **Other comments:** Do not refrigerate reconstituted vial as ganciclovir will crystallise out.	**Y-site compatible (but see Section A, 2.6):** fluconazole **Incompatible:** foscarnet

122

Formulation	Method	Dilution	Rate	Comments	Compatibility
Gelofusine					
(succinylated gelatin 4%) Bottle 500mL	(I) IV infusion. For rapid administration, a blood administration set can be used.		Dependent on patient's need. **Acute blood loss:** 500mL can be given in 5–10 minutes.	**Acute events that may accompany administration:** Severe anaphylactic reactions may occur. Transient increase in bleeding time may occur. **pH:** 7.4 **Flush:** N/S **Sodium content:** 77mmol/500mL **Other comments:** When given quickly warm bottle to not more than 37°C if possible. Discard unused bottle once seal has been opened.	**Y-site compatible (but see Section A, 2.6):** blood

- For abbreviations used in the Table, see Section A, 2.4.
  e.g. (C) IV = continuous intravenous infusion; (I) IV = intermittent intravenous infusion.
- Prepare a fresh infusion every 24hours unless otherwise specified.
- Presume suitability as single-use only unless otherwise specified.
- Always check with additional reference sources regarding compatibility information – see Section A, 2.2.

Formulation	Method	Dilution	Rate	Comments	Compatibility
Gentamicin					
Ampoule 20mg/2mL, 80mg/2mL	(I) IV infusion, once daily dosing	Dilute with 100mL N/S, G or G/S.	1 hour	**Acute events that may accompany administration:** Extravasation may cause tissue damage; for management guidelines, see Section A, 7. **pH:** 3–5 **Flush:** N/S **Sodium content:** Negligible **Other comments:** Plasma level monitoring is required	**Y-site compatible (but see Section A, 2.6):** aciclovir, amiodarone, atracurium, ciprofloxacin, clarithromycin, esmolol, fluconazole, foscarnet, insulin (soluble), labetalol, lorazepam, magnesium sulphate, meropenem, metronidazole, midazolam, pancuronium, vecuronium, zidovudine.

Formulation	Method	Dilution	Rate	Comments	Compatibility
	IV bolus	Dilution is not normally necessary but may be diluted with N/S (usually 10–20mL).	3–5 minutes		**Incompatible:** amoxicillin, amphotericin, azlocillin, benzylpenicillin, cephalosporins, chloramphenicol, co-amoxiclav, erythromycin, flucloxacillin, furosemide, heparin, eloHAES (hexastarch), penicillins, piperacillin/tazobactam, propofol, sodium bicarbonate, sulfadiazine.
	IM	Ready diluted.			

- For abbreviations used in the Table, see Section A, 2.4.
  e.g. (C) IV = continuous intravenous infusion; (I) IV = intermittent intravenous infusion.
- Prepare a fresh infusion every 24 hours unless otherwise specified.
- Presume suitability as single-use only unless otherwise specified.
- Always check with additional reference sources regarding compatibility information – see Section A, 2.2.

125

Formulation	Method	Dilution	Rate	Comments	Compatibility
Glucagon					
Vial 1 unit (1 mg)	IV bolus	Reconstitute with diluent provided to a concentration of 1 unit/1 mL (1 mg/mL). Do not dilute further.	3–5 minutes.	**Acute events that may accompany administration:** Hypotension (monitor blood pressure), vomiting, hypocalcaemia, hypokalaemia, hyperglycaemia. Extravasation may cause tissue damage; for management guidelines, see Section A, 7. **pH:** 2.5–3.5 **Flush:** G or N/S **Other comments:** Rarely, the unreconstituted medicine may show signs of fibril formation or may contain insoluble matter. If so, discard.	
	(C) IV infusion (unlicensed) for cardiogenic shock following β-blocker overdose. Give via a syringe or volumetric infusion pump.	Reconstitute vial with diluent provided (if using more than 2 units [2 mg], reconstitute with G to avoid administration of large amounts of preservative). Dilute with G to a convenient volume.	The airway must be protected in case of vomiting.		
	IM or S/C	Reconstitute vial with diluent provided.			

126

Formulation	Method	Dilution	Rate	Comments	Compatibility
Glucose					
5% (0.05 g/1 mL) – 100 mL, 250 mL, 500 mL, 1000 mL. 10% (0.1 g/1 mL) – 500 mL, 1000 mL 15% (0.15 g/1 mL) – 500 mL. 20%	IV bolus	Glucose infusions may be diluted with W if the concentration required is unavailable.	Usually up to 0.5 g/kg per hour will not cause glycosuria. Max. rate should generally not exceed 0.8 g/kg per hour	**Acute events that may accompany administration:** Hyperglycaemia, monitor blood glucose. Fluid overload and electrolyte dilution in congestive conditions. Infusion too quickly may cause local pain and venous irritation. Extravasation may cause tissue damage; for management guidelines, see Section A, 7. If G 10% is administered peripherally use a large vein and preferably alter the injection site daily. Concentrations >20% may cause venous irritation and thrombophlebitis if infused peripherally. Central administration is preferable. **pH:** G pH 4–4.2 Glucose concentrations >5%: pH 4–6 **Flush:** G or N/S	Check under individual medicine.
(0.2 g/1 mL) – 500 mL. 40% (0.4 g/1 mL) – 500 mL. 50% (0.5 g/1 mL) – 50 mL, 500 mL.	(C) IV or (I) IV infusion IV bolus 50% peripherally into a large vein. Emergency use only	As above.	When administered rapidly for hypoglycaemia give over 1–2 minutes		

- For abbreviations used in the Table, see Section A, 2.4.

  e.g. (C) IV = continuous intravenous infusion; (I) IV = intermittent intravenous infusion.
- Prepare a fresh infusion every 24 hours unless otherwise specified.
- Presume suitability as single-use only unless otherwise specified.
- Always check with additional reference sources regarding compatibility information – see Section A, 2.2.

127

Formulation	Method	Dilution	Rate	Comments	Compatibility
Glyceryl trinitrate					
Ampoule 50mg/10mL	(C) IV infusion Use a non-PVC giving set and syringe to prevent loss of medicine.	Dilute with N/S or G to a usual concentration of 1mg/1mL. Concentrations of up to 4mg/1mL have been used. **Paediatric information:** dilute 1mL of the 50mg/10mL solution to 50mL with N/S or G to give a concentration of 100 micrograms/ 1mL.	Titrate according to response. Rate control recommended.	**Acute events that may accompany administration:** Hypotension, monitor blood pressure. Tachycardia and paradoxical bradycardia which can lead to syncope and collapse, monitor heart rate. Nausea and retching. **pH:** 3.5–6.5 **Flush:** N/S **Other comments:** Contains ethanol and propylene glycol.	**Y-site compatible (but see Section A, 2.6):** aminophylline, amiodarone, atracurium, dobutamine, dopamine, furosemide, heparin, insulin (soluble), lidocaine, magnesium sulphate, ranitidine, sodium nitroprusside, streptokinase. **Incompatible:** alteplase, hydralazine.

Formulation	Method	Dilution	Rate	Comments	Compatibility
Glycopyrronium					
Ampoule 200 micrograms/ 1 mL, 600 micrograms/3 mL	IV bolus	May be diluted with N/S, G/S or G.	Rapidly	**Acute events that may accompany administration:** Arrhythmias, monitor heart rate. Extravasation may cause tissue damage; for management guidelines, see Section A, 7. **pH:** 2.3–4.3 **Flush:** N/S or G **Sodium content:** 0.15 mmol/1 mL	**Incompatible:** alkaline medicines, e.g. aminophylline, azathioprine, co-trimoxazole, dantrolene, epoprostenol, furosemide, ganciclovir, omeprazole, phenobarbital, thiopental.
	IM or S/C (s/c unlicensed)				
	(C) S/C infusion (unlicensed)	May dilute with N/S, G/S or G.			

- For abbreviations used in the Table, see Section A, 2.4.
- e.g. (C) IV = continuous intravenous infusion; (I) IV = intermittent intravenous infusion.
- Prepare a fresh infusion every 24 hours unless otherwise specified.
- Presume suitability as single-use only unless otherwise specified.
- Always check with additional reference sources regarding compatibility information – see Section A, 2.2.

129

Formulation	Method	Dilution	Rate	Comments	Compatibility
Glycopyrronium and neostigmine					
(500 micrograms and 2.5 mg) Ampoule 1 mL	IV bolus	May dilute with W or N/S.	1–2 mL over 10–30 seconds.	**Acute events that may accompany administration:** Bronchospasm, arrhythmias and bradycardia; monitor heart rate. **pH:** 3.4–4.1 **Flush:** N/S or G **Other comments:** irritation may develop after skin contact. May be absorbed through the skin. Wash affected area with soap and water.	Do not infuse with other medicines.
Gonadorelin (gonadotrophin-releasing hormone or GnRH; LH-RH)					
Vial 100 micrograms (HRF)	IV bolus (for pituitary function test)	Reconstitute the 100 microgram vial with the 1 mL diluent provided.	Few seconds.	**pH:** 4–8 **Flush:** N/S	

Formulation	Method	Dilution	Rate	Comments	Compatibility
Granisetron					
Ampoule 1 mg/1 mL, 3 mg/3 mL	IV bolus	Dilute each 1 mg to 5 mL and 3 mg to 15 mL with N/S.	Min. 30 seconds.	**pH:** 5–7 **Flush:** N/S **Sodium content:** 1.17 mmol/3 mg	**Y-site compatible (but see Section A, 2.6):** dexamethasone, mannitol 10%.
		Paediatrics: dilute appropriate dose to 10–30 mL with N/S, G or G/S.	Min. 5 minutes.		
	(C) S/C infusion (unlicensed) via syringe pump	May be used undiluted or diluted with N/S or G.			

- For abbreviations used in the Table, see Section A, 2.4.
  e.g. (C) IV = continuous intravenous infusion; (I) IV = intermittent intravenous infusion.
- Prepare a fresh infusion every 24 hours unless otherwise specified.
- Presume suitability as single-use only unless otherwise specified.
- Always check with additional reference sources regarding compatibility information – see Section A, 2.2.

131

Formulation	Method	Dilution	Rate	Comments	Compatibility
Haloperidol lactate					
Ampoule 5mg/1mL, 10mg/2mL, 20mg/2mL	IV bolus	May be diluted with N/S (concentration prepared must not exceed 500 micrograms in 1mL) or G.	1–2 minutes, longer if possible. Max. rate 5mg/ minute.	**Acute events that may accompany administration:** Rapid administration may cause severe hypotension and tachycardia. Monitor blood pressure and heart rate. Extravasation may cause tissue damage; for management guidelines, see Section A, 7. **pH:** 3–3.8 **Flush:** N/S or G **Sodium content:** Negligible **Paediatric information:** Avoid IV administration.	**Compatibility in S/C syringe pump:** with diamorphine; see Section A, 8 for details. **Y-site compatible (but see Section A, 2.6):** dobutamine, dopamine, G, lorazepam, midazolam, ondansetron, propofol, remifentanil. **Incompatible:** amphotericin, fluconazole, foscarnet, heparin, piperacillin/tazobactam.
	(C) IV infusion (unlicensed ICU practice) via syringe pump	Dilute to a suitable volume with G (e.g. 30mg in 50mL).			
	IM	Ready diluted.			
	S/C (unlicensed) or (C) S/C infusion via syringe pump	Ready diluted. But see dilution recommendations above.			

Formulation	Method	Dilution	Rate	Comments	Compatibility
Heparin sodium					
Ampoule 1000 units/ 1 mL, 5000 units/1 mL, 25,000 units/ 1 mL, 50 units/ 5 mL N/S. Infusion bag 500 units in 500mL N/S	(C) IV infusion (preferred method) via syringe pump	Dilute required dose with N/S, G or G/S to a convenient volume (25–50mL is usually used). When adding heparin to an IV fluid the container should be inverted at least six times to prevent pooling.		**Acute events that may accompany administration: Skin necrosis** contraindicates further use of heparin. **pH:** 5–8 **Flush:** N/S **Sodium content:** Negligible **Other comments:** Calcium or sodium heparin may be used subcutaneously. Inject into the lateral abdominal wall using a 26-gauge needle. Insert needle perpendicularly into a pinched fold of skin. Do not rub site of injection.	**Y-site compatible (but see Section A, 2.6):** aciclovir, adrenaline (epinephrine), aminophylline, atracurium, atropine, benzylpenicillin, calcium salts, cefotaxime, ceftazidime, ceftriaxone, cefuroxime, clindamycin, dexamethasone, digoxin, dopamine, fentanyl, flucloxacillin, fluconazole, fosarnet, furosemide, hydralazine, insulin (soluble), labetalol, lidocaine, lorazepam, magnesium sulphate, meropenem, metoclopramide, metronidazole, midazolam, neostigmine, noradrenaline

Heparin sodium cont'd from p. 134 overleaf

- For abbreviations used in the Table, see Section A, 2.4.
  e.g. (C) IV = continuous intravenous infusion; (I) IV = intermittent intravenous infusion.
- Prepare a fresh infusion every 24 hours unless otherwise specified.
- Presume suitability as single-use only unless otherwise specified.
- Always check with additional reference sources regarding compatibility information – see Section A, 2.2.

Heparin sodium cont'd from p. 133

Formulation	Method	Dilution	Rate	Comments	Compatibility
	IV bolus	Ready diluted.	3–5 minutes		(norepinephrine), ondansetron, pancuronium, piperacillin/ tazobactam, potassium chloride, procainamide, propofol, propranolol, ranitidine, sodium bicarbonate, sodium nitroprusside, remifentanil, streptokinase, suxamethonium, thiopental, vecuronium, zidovudine. **Incompatible:** ciprofloxacin, clarithromycin, gentamicin, haloperidol, phenytoin, vancomycin.
	S/C	Ready diluted.			
Heparin calcium					
Prefilled syringe 5000 units/ 0.2mL, 20000 units/ 0.8mL	S/C			Inject into the lateral abdominal wall using a 26-gauge needle. Insert needle perpendicularly into a pinched fold of skin. Do not rub site of injection.	

Formulation	Method	Dilution	Rate	Comments	Compatibility
Hydralazine					
Ampoule 20mg	Slow IV bolus	Reconstitute with 1mL W, then dilute to 10mL with N/S.	Over 2–3 minutes, may be repeated after 20–30 minutes.	**Acute events that may accompany administration:** Tachycardia, hypotension, monitor blood pressure and heart rate. Extravasation may cause tissue damage; for management guidelines, see Section A, 7. **pH:** 3.5–4.2 **Flush:** N/S.	**Y-site compatible (but see Section A, 2.6):** heparin, hydrocortisone sodium succinate, potassium chloride. **Incompatible:** G, aminophylline, furosemide glyceryl trinitrate, sulphonamides. Hydralazine is unstable in alkaline solutions.
	(C) IV infusion via volumetric pump	Reconstitute as above then dilute to 500mL with N/S.	**Adults:** Initially 200–300 micrograms/minute. Maintenance 50–150 micrograms/ minute.	**Sodium content:** Nil **Displacement:** Negligible	
	(C) IV infusion via syringe pump	Reconstitute three ampoules with 1ml W each and further dilute to 60mL with N/S (local practice).			
	IM (unlicensed)	Reconstitute with 1mL W.			

- For abbreviations used in the Table, see Section A, 2.4.

  e.g. (C) IV = continuous intravenous infusion; (I) IV = intermittent intravenous infusion.
- Prepare a fresh infusion every 24hours unless otherwise specified.
- Presume suitability as single-use only unless otherwise specified.
- Always check with additional reference sources regarding compatibility information – see Section A, 2.2.

135

Formulation	Method	Dilution	Rate	Comments	Compatibility
Hydrocortisone sodium succinate					
Vial 100 mg	IV bolus	Reconstitute with 2 ml W. May be diluted with N/S, G or G/S.	Min. 1–10 minutes.	**Acute events that may accompany administration:** Hypotension, cyanosis. **pH:** 7–8 **Flush:** N/S, G **Sodium content:** 0.5 mmol/100 mg	**Y-site compatible (but see Section A, 2.6):** aciclovir, adrenaline (epinephrine), aminophylline, atracurium, calcium gluconate, chloramphenicol, daunorubicin, dexamethasone, digoxin, dopamine, fentanyl, foscarnet, furosemide, hydralazine, insulin (soluble), lidocaine, lorazepam, magnesium sulphate, morphine, noradrenaline (norepinephrine), ondansetron, paclitaxel, pancuronium, piperacillin/ tazobactam, potassium chloride, propofol, sodium bicarbonate, vecuronium. **Incompatible:** ciprofloxacin, heparin, midazolam, phenytoin.
	(I) IV infusion	Reconstitute as above then dilute to a maximum concentration of 1 mg/1 mL with N/S, G, or G/S.	20–30 minutes.		
	IM	Reconstitute with 2 mL W.			

Formulation	Method	Dilution	Rate	Comments	Compatibility
Hyoscine butylbromide					
Ampoule 20 mg/1 mL	IV bolus	May be diluted with G or N/S.	3–5 minutes.	Extravasation may cause tissue damage; for management guidelines, see Section A, 7. **pH:** 3.7–5.5 **Flush:** N/S or G **Sodium content:** 0.4 mmol/1 mL	**Compatibility in S/C syringe pump:** for diamorphine see Section A, 8 for details. **Y-site compatible (but see Section A, 2.6):** most aqueous radiological contrast media, diamorphine, morphine, pethidine.
	IM	Ready diluted.			
	(C) S/C infusion via syringe pump	May be diluted with G or N/S.			

- For abbreviations used in the Table, see Section A, 2.4.
e.g. (C) IV = continuous intravenous infusion; (I) IV = intermittent intravenous infusion.
- Prepare a fresh infusion every 24 hours unless otherwise specified.
- Presume suitability as single-use only unless otherwise specified.
- Always check with additional reference sources regarding compatibility information – see Section A, 2.2.

Formulation	Method	Dilution	Rate	Comments	Compatibility
Hyoscine hydrobromide					
Ampoule 400 micrograms/1mL, 600 micrograms/ 1 mL	IV bolus (for acute use only)	May be diluted with W.		**Acute events that may accompany administration:** Bradycardia can occur following low doses. Drowsiness leading to coma (CNS stimulation may precede CNS depression). Toxic doses can cause hyperpyrexia, respiratory depression and rapid respiration. Monitor heart rate, temperature, respiration and sedation level. **pH:** 5–7 **Flush:** N/S **Sodium content:** Negligible	**Compatibility in S/C syringe pump:** for diamorphine, see Section A, 8 for details.
	S/C injection or (C) S/C infusion	Infusion may be diluted with W.			
	IM	Ready diluted.			

Formulation	Method	Dilution	Rate	Comments	Compatibility
Ibuprofen					
5 mg/mL injection 2 mL	IV infusion	Preferably undiluted. Can be diluted with N/S or G.	Over 15 minutes.	**Acute events that may accompany administration:** Necrotising enterocolitis, intestinal perforation, haemorrhage, ischaemic brain injury, fluid retention and oliguria. **pH:** 7.8–8.2 **Flush:** G or N/S **Sodium content:** 0.25 mmol	Do not infuse with other medicines.
Iloprost (unlicensed)					
Ampoule 100 micrograms/ 1 mL (100 micrograms = 100000 nanograms)	(I) IV infusion via a syringe pump	Dilute each ampoule to 50 mL N/S or G.	Commence at 0.5 nanograms/ kg per minute. Increase dose in increments of 0.5 nanograms/ kg per minute every 15–30 minutes to a max. of 2 nanograms/kg per minute. Usual total duration of infusion is 6 hours.	**Acute events that may accompany administration:** Hypotension, tachycardia, arrhythmia, extrasystole, nausea and vomiting. Monitor blood pressure and heart rate every 30 minutes. Stop infusion if side effects occur. Wait 1 hour and recommence at half previous rate. **pH:** 7.8–8.8 **Flush:** N/S or G **Sodium content:** 0.15 mmol/ampoule Contains ethanol.	Do not infuse with other medicines.

- For abbreviations used in the Table, see Section A, 2.4.
  e.g. (C) IV = continuous intravenous infusion; (I) IV = intermittent intravenous infusion.
- Prepare a fresh infusion every 24 hours unless otherwise specified.
- Presume suitability as single-use only unless otherwise specified.
- Always check with additional reference sources regarding compatibility information – see Section A, 2.2.

Formulation	Method	Dilution	Rate	Comments	Compatibility
Imipenem with cilastatin					
Vial 500mg containing imipenem 500mg with cilastatin 500mg (Primaxin for intravenous infusion)	(I) IV infusion (IM formulation not suitable for IV use)	Reconstitute 500mg with 100mL N/S, G or G/S. Fluid restriction: 500mg in 60mL.	**Adults:** doses up to 250–500mg over 20–30 minutes; 1g over 40–60 minutes.	**Acute events that may accompany administration:** Erythema, local pain and induration, thrombophlebitis. Slow infusion rate in patients who develop nausea. **pH:** 6.5–7.5 **Flush:** N/S, G or G/S **Sodium content:** 1.72mmol/vial **Displacement:** Negligible **Other comments:** Stable for 3 hours at room temperature or 24 hours in a refrigerator after reconstitution with specified diluents.	**Y-site compatible (but see Section A, 2.6):** aciclovir, foscarnet, insulin (soluble), ondansetron, propofol. **Incompatible:** fluconazole, lorazepam, midazolam, pethidine, sodium bicarbonate.
	IM injection (IV formulation not suitable for IM use)	Give by deep IM injection into a large muscle mass (such as the gluteal muscle or lateral part of the thigh).			

Formulation	Method	Dilution	Rate	Comments	Compatibility
Indometacin (indomethacin)					
Vial 1 mg	(I) IV infusion via syringe pump	Reconstitute with 1–2 mL N/S or W. Further dilution not recommended.	20–30 minutes.	**Acute events that may accompany administration:** Monitor for bleeding **pH:** 6–7.5 (indometacin is not buffered and reconstitution at pH levels <6 may cause precipitation of insoluble indometacin). **Flush:** N/S **Sodium content:** Negligible **Displacement:** Negligible **Other comments:** Discard solution if cloudy.	**Incompatible:** G. Do not infuse with other medicines.

- For abbreviations used in the Table, see Section A, 2.4.
- e.g. (C) IV = continuous intravenous infusion; (I) IV = intermittent intravenous infusion.
- Prepare a fresh infusion every 24 hours unless otherwise specified.
- Presume suitability as single-use only unless otherwise specified.
- Always check with additional reference sources regarding compatibility information – see Section A, 2.2.

Formulation	Method	Dilution	Rate	Comments	Compatibility
Infliximab					
Vial 100mg	(I) IV infusion	Reconstitute each vial with 10mL of W. Gently swirl to dissolve the lysophilised powder. DO NOT SHAKE. Allow the reconstituted solution to stand for 5 minutes. Dilute the total volume of the reconstituted solution dose to 250mL with N/S.	2 hours.	**Acute events that may accompany administration:** Monitor patient for 2 hours post-infusion; anaphylaxis equipment and medicines must be available (adrenaline [epinephrine], antihistamines, corticosteroids and an artificial airway). Patients may be pre-treated with an antihistamine, hydrocortisone and/or paracetamol to reduce the risk of infusion-related events, especially if a previous reaction has been noted. **pH:** 7.2 **Flush:** N/S **Sodium content:** 8.3mg/vial **Displacement:** Negligible **Other comments:** After reconstitution vials maybe stored for up to 3 hours at room temperature. Diluted solutions are stable for up to 24 hours when stored at 2–8°C. Do not store any unused portions for reuse.	Do not infuse with other medicines.

Formulation	Method	Dilution	Rate	Comments	Compatibility
Insulin (human soluble) (Actrapid human)					
Vial 100 units/mL 10mL Penfill 300 units/3mL Pen 300 units/3mL	IV bolus	Ready diluted.	3–5 minutes.	**Acute events that may accompany administration:** Hypoglycaemia: monitor blood glucose. **pH:** Neutral (6.6–8) **Flush:** N/S or G **Other comments:** Loss of medicine into bag, plastic syringe or giving set may occur. When adding insulin to bag, ensure that insulin is not injected into dead space of injection port of infusion bag. When preparing an infusion, flush giving set with 50mL of the infusion to saturate the PVC of the line.	**Y-site compatible (but see Section A, 2.6):** amiodarone, clarithromycin, dobutamine, dopamine, gentamicin, glyceryl trinitrate, heparin sodium, hydrocortisone sodium succinate, magnesium sulphate, morphine, pethidine, potassium chloride, propofol, sodium nitroprusside, sodium bicarbonate, terbutaline, vancomycin. **Incompatible:** aminophylline, calcium, co-trimoxazole and other sulphonamides, dopamine, magnesium, noradrenaline (norepinephrine), phenytoin, thiopental, zinc.
	(C) IV infusion. Syringe pump recommended.	Dilute in syringe with N/S to 1 unit/1mL.	Titrate rate to keep blood glucose in the target range (e.g. 4–8mmol/L).		
	(C) IV infusion via volumetric pump (GKI regimen). Used occasionally in minor elective surgery in patients with diabetes.	Typically 10–15 units insulin and 10mmol potassium chloride added to 500mL G 10%. The concentration of insulin may be increased or decreased by 2–4 units in each 500mL G 10% to maintain blood glucose levels in the range 4–8mmol/L, as clinically indicated.	100mL/hour.		
	IM or S/C	Ready diluted.			

- For abbreviations used in the Table, see Section A, 2.4.
  e.g. (C) IV = continuous intravenous infusion; (I) IV = intermittent intravenous infusion.
- Prepare a fresh infusion every 24hours unless otherwise specified.
- Presume suitability as single-use only unless otherwise specified.
- Always check with additional reference sources regarding compatibility information – see Section A, 2.2.

Formulation	Method	Dilution	Rate	Comments	Compatibility
Iron sucrose complex (Venofer)					
Ampoule 100mg/5mL of elemental iron	(I) IV infusion via volumetric infusion pump	Dilute dose up to 1mg/1mL N/S (typically in 100mL).	Initial rate: 25mg over the first 15 minutes. Titrate upwards over next 30 minutes according to patient tolerance. Max. rate: 3.33mg/minute (or 200mg/hour if diluted in 100mL).	**Acute events that may accompany administration: Anaphylaxis:** have resuscitation equipment available. Administer hydrocortisone 100mg IV and ibuprofen 200mg PO immediately before dose. Extravasation may cause tissue damage see Section A, 7 for details. Nursing observations are required every 15 minutes. The higher the dose the greater the risk of side effects. **pH:** strongly alkaline **Flush:** N/S **Other comments:** Do not use ampoules if any sediment is present. A slower infusion rate may improve patient intolerance.	Do not infuse with other medicines.

144

Formulation	Method	Dilution	Rate	Comments	Compatibility
Isoniazid					
Ampoule 50mg/2mL	IV bolus	Ready diluted.	3–5 minutes.	**pH:** 5.6–6 **Flush:** N/S **Other comments:** also licensed for intrapleural and intrathecal administration.	**Incompatible:** glucose solutions.
	IM	Ready diluted.			
Isoprenaline (available on special order only)					
Ampoule 2mg/2mL, Min-I-Jet 200 micrograms/ 10mL	(C) IV infusion with a volumetric infusion pump preferably via a central line.	Dilute with G (adults: usually to 500mL).	Adjust rate according to response and indication.	**Acute events that may accompany administration:** May precipitate ventricular extrasystoles and arrhythmias. If heart rate >100 beats/minute or if premature heart beats or changes in **ECG** develop consider slowing or stopping infusion. Should be given only in specialist units with invasive haemodynamic monitoring. Extravasation may cause tissue damage; for management guidelines, see Section A, 7. **pH:** 2.5–4.2 (pH of final infusion must remain <5 to avoid decomposition of the medicine). **Flush:** G, N/S	**Y-site compatible (but see Section A, 2.6):** amiodarone, atracurium, calcium chloride, dobutamine, dopamine, heparin, hydralazine, magnesium sulphate, sodium nitroprusside, noradrenaline (norepinephrine), pancuronium, potassium chloride, vecuronium, verapamil. **Incompatible:** aminophylline, furosemide, sodium bicarbonate.
	IV bolus	Ready diluted.	3–5 minutes.		

- For abbreviations used in the Table, see Section A, 2.4.
  e.g. (C) IV = continuous intravenous infusion; (I) IV = intermittent intravenous infusion.
- Prepare a fresh infusion every 24 hours unless otherwise specified.
- Presume suitability as single-use only unless otherwise specified.
- Always check with additional reference sources regarding compatibility information – see Section A, 2.2.

Formulation	Method	Dilution	Rate	Comments	Compatibility
Itraconazole					
Vial 250 mg/25 mL (+50 mL N/S infusion bag provided)	(I) IV infusion	Add the whole volume (25 mL) of the itraconazole vial to the bag of N/S provided. The bag now contains 250 mg itraconazole in 75 mL (3.33 mg/mL), e.g. to give a 200 mg dose, administer 60 mL only. Use a 0.2 μm in-line filter.	60 minutes.	**pH:** 4.5–5.2 **Flush:** N/S **Sodium content:** Negligible **Displacement:** N/A **Other comments:** Risk of accumulation of excipient (hydroxypropyl-β-cyclodextrin) in renal failure. Patients with renal impairment defined as creatinine clearance <30 mL/minute should not be treated with intravenous itraconazole.	Itraconazole has the potential to precipitate when diluted in solutions other than the 50 ml N/S injection supplied.

146

Formulation	Method	Dilution	Rate	Comments	Compatibility
Ketamine					
Vial 200mg/20mL, 500mg/5mL, 1000mg/10mL	IV bolus	Ready diluted.	Min. 60 seconds.	**Acute events that may accompany administration:** Temporary elevation of blood pressure and heart rate frequently occur (about 25% increase in baseline blood pressure). Also arrhythmias, laryngospasm, respiratory depression and hypotension. Tonic and clonic movements resembling seizures may occur but are not an indication for adjusting therapy. Hallucinations and psychotic sequelae. Extravasation may cause tissue damage; for management guidelines, see Section A, 7. **pH:** 3.5–5.5 **Flush:** N/S or G **Sodium content:** Negligible	**Compatibility in S/C syringe pump:** with diamorphine, see Section A, 8, for details. Also compatible with lidocaine (local practice). **Y-site compatible (but see Section A, 2.6):** midazolam, morphine **Incompatible:** barbiturates, doxapram
	(C) IV infusion via volumetric infusion or syringe pump.	Dilute to 1mg/1mL with G or N/S. In fluid restriction dilute to a maximum concentration of 50mg/1mL (unlicensed).	Dependent on indication; see package insert for details.		
	(C) S/C infusion via syringe pump (unlicensed)	Dilute with N/S.			

- For abbreviations used in the Table, see Section A, 2.4.
  e.g. (C) IV = continuous intravenous infusion; (I) IV = intermittent intravenous infusion.
- Prepare a fresh infusion every 24 hours unless otherwise specified.
- Presume suitability as single-use only unless otherwise specified.
- Always check with additional reference sources regarding compatibility information – see Section A, 2.2.

147

Formulation	Method	Dilution	Rate	Comments	Compatibility
Ketorolac					
Ampoule 10mg/1mL	IV bolus	May be diluted with N/S or G.	Min. 15 seconds.	**Acute events that may accompany administration:** Anaphylaxis, bradycardia and flushing. Monitor blood pressure and heart rate. **pH:** 6.9–7.9 **Flush:** N/S or G **Other comments:** Only licensed for use on up to 2 consecutive days.	**Compatibility in S/C syringe pump:** with diamorphine, see Section A, 8 for detail. **Incompatible:** haloperidol, hydroxyzine, morphine, pethidine, promethazine.
	IM	Ready diluted.			
	(C) S/C infusion via syringe pump (unlicensed)	May be diluted with W.			
Labetalol					
Ampoule 100mg/20mL	IV bolus	Ready diluted.	Maximum rate. 50mg/minute can be repeated every 5 minutes to a maximum dose of 200mg.	**Acute events that may accompany administration:** Bradycardia. ECG monitoring recommended. Hypotension, monitor blood pressure; the patient should remain supine for more than 3 hours after administration. Extravasation may cause tissue damage; for management guidelines, see Section A, 7. **pH:** 3.5–4.2 **Flush:** N/S **Sodium content:** Negligible	**Y-site compatible (but see Section A, 2.6):** dopamine, gentamicin, heparin, magnesium sulphate, morphine, pethidine, potassium chloride, ranitidine. **Incompatible:** sodium bicarbonate.
	(C) IV infusion via volumetric infusion	Dilute to 1mg/1mL with G/S or G. ICU practice: undiluted.	Usual maximum rate 2mg/minute.		

148

Formulation	Method	Dilution	Rate	Comments	Compatibility
Lenograstim					
Vial 105 micrograms (13.4MU), 263 micrograms (33.6MU)	S/C	Reconstitute each vial with 1mL W provided. Mix gently until dissolved. Do not shake vigorously.		**Acute events that may accompany administration:** Pain at injection site when given S/C. More likely to occur if vial is taken straight out of fridge before administration. **pH:** 6.5 **Flush:** N/S **Sodium content:** Negligible	
	(I) IV infusion	Reconstitute as above then dilute with up to 50mL N/S for each vial of Granocyte-13 or up to 100mL N/S for Granocyte-34.	30 minutes.		

- For abbreviations used in the Table, see Section A, 2.4.
  - e.g. (C) IV = continuous intravenous infusion; (I) IV = intermittent intravenous infusion.
  - Prepare a fresh infusion every 24 hours unless otherwise specified.
  - Presume suitability as single-use only unless otherwise specified.
  - Always check with additional reference sources regarding compatibility information – see Section A, 2.2.

Formulation	Method	Dilution	Rate	Comments	Compatibility
Levomepromazine (Methotrimeprazine)					
Ampoule 25 mg/1 mL	IV bolus	Dilute with at least an equal volume of N/S before administration.	3–5 minutes.	**Acute events that may accompany administration:** Postural hypotension particularly in patients over 50 years; monitor blood pressure. **Other comments:** Discard infusion if pink or yellow coloration occurs. **pH:** 4.5 **Flush:** N/S **Sodium content:** Negligible	**Compatibility in S/C syringe pump:** with diamorphine, see Section A, 8 for details. **Incompatible:** alkaline agents, heparin, ranitidine.
	IM	Ready diluted.			
	(C) S/C via syringe pump	Dilute with a suitable volume of W (local practice) or N/S.			

Formulation	Method	Dilution	Rate	Comments	Compatibility
Lidocaine (lignocaine)					
Min-I-Jet 1% (100 mg/ 10 mL), Infusion bag: 0.1% (1 mg/mL), 0.2% (2 mg/ mL), 0.4% (4 mg/mL) in G 500 mL. Ampoule: 0.5% (100 mg/ 20 mL), 1% (20 mg/2 mL, 50 mg/5 mL), 2% (40 mg/ 2 mL, 100 mg/5 mL, 200 mg/10 mL, 400 mg/20 mL)	IV bolus (initial loading dose followed by infusion)		**Adults:** usual maximum rate 50 mg/minute. If an intravenous infusion is not immediately available the initial IV bolus of 50–100 mg can be repeated if necessary once or twice at intervals of not less than 10 minutes	**Acute events that may accompany administration:** Rapid administration may produce dizziness, paraesthesia and drowsiness. Hypotension and tachycardia leading to arrest, **ECG** monitoring required. CNS and peripheral reactions are dose related. Extravasation may cause tissue damage; for management guidelines, see Section A, 7. **pH:** 3.5–6 (pre-mixed infusion), 5–7 (Min-I-Jet) **Flush:** N/S **Sodium content:** Variable	**Y-site compatible (but see Section A, 2.6):** Adrenaline (epinephrine), alteplase, aminophylline, amiodarone, bretylium, calcium chloride, calcium gluconate, cefuroxime, ciprofloxacin, dexamethasone, digoxin, dopamine, dobutamine, erythromycin, flucloxacillin, furosemide, gentamicin, glyceryl trinitrate, heparin, hydralazine, hydrocortisone sodium succinate, insulin (soluble), isoprenaline, morphine,

Lidocaine (lignocaine) cont'd on p. 152 overleaf

Lidocaine (lignocaine) cont'd on p. 152 overleaf

- For abbreviations used in the Table, see Section A, 2.4.
- e.g. (C) IV = continuous intravenous infusion; (I) IV = intermittent intravenous infusion.
- Prepare a fresh infusion every 24 hours unless otherwise specified.
- Presume suitability as single-use only unless otherwise specified.
- Always check with additional reference sources regarding compatibility information – see Section A, 2.2.

Lidocaine (lignocaine) cont'd from p. 151

Formulation	Method	Dilution	Rate	Comments	Compatibility
	(C) IV infusion via volumetric infusion pump	Dilute with G to suggested concentration of 0.1–0.4% (1–4 mg/mL). Use ready prepared solutions where possible.	**Adults:** maximum rate 4 mg/minute		noradrenaline (norepinephrine), pethidine, phenylephrine, potassium chloride, procainamide, sodium bicarbonate, sodium nitroprusside, streptokinase, verapamil. **Incompatible:** phenytoin

152

Formulation	Method	Dilution	Rate	Comments	Compatibility
Linezolid					
Infusion bag 600 mg/300 mL	(I) IV infusion	Ready-made infusion bag	30–120 minutes.	**Acute events that may accompany administration:** Injection site pain, phlebitis, thrombophlebitis. **pH:** 5.6–6.4 **Flush:** N/S **Sodium content:** 5 mmol/bag **Displacement:** N/A **Other comments:** G content: 13.7 g/300 mL. Take into account patients with diabetes mellitus or other conditions associated with G intolerance.	**Incompatible:** amphotericin B, chlorpromazine hydrochloride, diazepam, pentamidine isothionate, erythromycin lactobionate, phenytoin sodium, sulfamethoxazole/ trimethoprim, ceftriaxone.
Liothyronine					
Ampoule 20 micrograms	IV bolus	Reconstitute with 1–2 mL W	3–5 minutes.	**Acute events that may accompany administration:** Arrhythmias, tachycardia, palpitation and cramp in skeletal muscle; monitor pulse. Extravasation may cause tissue damage; for management guidelines, see Section A, 7. **pH:** 9.8–11.2 **Flush:** N/S **Sodium content:** Negligible	

- For abbreviations used in the Table, see Section A, 2.4.
  e.g. (C) IV = continuous intravenous infusion; (I) IV = intermittent intravenous infusion.
- Prepare a fresh infusion every 24 hours unless otherwise specified.
- Presume suitability as single-use only unless otherwise specified.
- Always check with additional reference sources regarding compatibility information – see Section A, 2.2.

Formulation	Method	Dilution	Rate	Comments	Compatibility
Lorazepam					
Ampoule 4 mg/1 mL	IV bolus. Avoid injecting into small veins	May be diluted up to 2 mL with N/S or W.	Usually 3–5 minutes. Maximum rate 2 mg/minute.	**Acute events that may accompany administration:** Rapid administration increases risk of respiratory depression and hypotension. Monitor blood pressure and respiratory rate. **Flush:** N/S	
	IM (use only when oral and intravenous routes not possible)	Dilute with 1 mL N/S or W.			

Formulation	Method	Dilution	Rate	Comments	Compatibility
Magnesium sulphate					
Ampoule 50% 1g/2mL, 5g/10mL containing 2.03mmol Mg²⁺/1mL	IV bolus	Dilute to a maximum concentration of 200mg/1mL with N/S, G/S or G.	3–5 minutes **Adults:** maximum rate 150mg/minute (or 0.6mmol Mg²⁺/minute).	**Acute events that may accompany administration:** Rapid administration may cause flushing and hypotension. In pregnancy blood pressure, respiratory rate, magnesium plasma levels and fluid monitoring are necessary and **ECG** monitoring is recommended. Extravasation may cause tissue damage; for management guidelines, see Section A, 7. **pH:** 5.5–8 **Flush:** N/S **Other comments:** Avoid injecting into small veins.	**Y-site compatible (but see Section A, 2.6):** amphotericin, calcium gluconate, co-trimoxazole, dobutamine, erythromycin, furosemide, glyceryl trinitrate, heparin, hydrocortisone sodium succinate, insulin (soluble), isoprenaline, labetalol, metronidazole, morphine, noradrenaline (norepinephrine), potassium chloride, streptokinase. **Incompatible:** alkaline agents, calcium salts, clindamycin, hydrocortisone sodium succinate, phosphates, sulphates.
	(I) IV infusion	Dilute each 1g (4mmol Mg²⁺) to a suitable volume (at least 10mL for peripheral use) with N/S, G/S or G. May be infused centrally at a concentration of 1–2mmol/1mL.	**Adults:** usual dose 1–2g/hour.		
	IM (in alternate buttocks)	**Adults:** doses may be diluted to 25%. **Children:** must be diluted to 20% in G or N/S.			

- For abbreviations used in the Table, see Section A, 2.4.
  e.g. (C) IV = continuous intravenous infusion; (I) IV = intermittent intravenous infusion.
- Prepare a fresh infusion every 24 hours unless otherwise specified.
- Presume suitability as single-use only unless otherwise specified.
- Always check with additional reference sources regarding compatibility information – see Section A, 2.2.

Formulation	Method	Dilution	Rate	Comments	Compatibility
Mannitol					
Infusion bag 10% (0.1 g/1 mL), 20% (0.2 g/1 mL), 500 mL	IV bolus – test dose	Ready diluted.	0.2 g/kg over 3–5 minutes.	**Acute events that may accompany administration:** Nausea, vomiting, thirst, headache, chills, fever, tachycardia, chest pain, hypo- or hypertension. Extravasation may cause tissue damage; for management guidelines, see Section A, 7. **pH:** 4.5–7 **Flush:** N/S or G **Other comments:** Central administration is preferred because extravasation can cause oedema, skin necrosis and thrombophlebitis. Use administration sets incorporating a filter for concentrations of 20%. Infusion may crystallise at low temperatures; redissolve by warming.	**Y-site compatible (but see Section A, 2.6):** cisplatin, fluorouracil, dopamine, granisetron, ondansetron, paclitaxel, potassium chloride (local practice). **Incompatible:** in strongly alkaline or acidic solutions.
	(C) IV infusion via volumetric pump preferably centrally.	Ready diluted.	**Adults:** 50–200 g over 24 hours.		

Formulation	Method	Dilution	Rate	Comments	Compatibility
Meropenem					
Vial 250 mg, 500 mg, 1 g	IV bolus	Reconstitute each 250 mg with 5 mL W. This produces an approximate concentration of 50 mg/1 mL. Fluid restriction: 1 g in 10 mL (anecdotal).	5 minutes.	**Acute events that may accompany administration:** Thrombophlebitis and rash. **pH:** 7.3–8.3 **Flush:** N/S or G **Sodium content:** 3.9 mmol/1 g **Displacement:** 0.22 mL/250 mg. Add 4.8 mL W to 250 mg vial to give a concentration of 50 mg/1 mL.	Do not infuse with other medicines.
	(I) IV infusion	Reconstitute as above and further dilute dose to 50–250 mL with N/S or G.	15–30 minutes.		

- For abbreviations used in the Table, see Section A, 2.4.
  e.g. (C) IV = continuous intravenous infusion; (I) IV = intermittent intravenous infusion.
- Prepare a fresh infusion every 24 hours unless otherwise specified.
- Presume suitability as single-use only unless otherwise specified.
- Always check with additional reference sources regarding compatibility information – see Section A, 2.2.

157

Formulation	Method	Dilution	Rate	Comments	Compatibility
Mesna					
Ampoule 400 mg/4 mL, 1000 mg/10 mL	(I) IV infusion	Dilute with a convenient volume of N/S or G.	15–30 minutes.	**Acute events that may accompany administration:** Nausea, vomiting, diarrhoea, fatigue, rash, hypotension, tachycardia. **pH:** 6.5–8.5 **Flush:** N/S **Sodium content:** About 6 mmol in 10 mL.	**Compatible in infusion bag (but see Section A, 2.6):** ifosfamide **Incompatible:** carboplatin, cisplatin
	IV bolus	Ready diluted.	3 minutes.		
	(C) IV infusion via volumetric infusion pump after (I) IV loading dose	Dilute with a convenient volume of N/S or G.	30 minutes to 24 hours.		

158

Formulation	Method	Dilution	Rate	Comments	Compatibility
Methylprednisolone sodium succinate					
Vial 40 mg, 125 mg, 500 mg, 1 g, 2 g	IV bolus (doses <250 mg)	Reconstitute with diluent provided.	Give slowly, min. 5 minutes.	**Acute events that may accompany administration:** Bradycardia, hypotension or hypertension and rarely anaphylaxis. If administered too quickly cardiac arrhythmias, circulatory collapse and cardiac arrest may occur. **pH:** 7.4–8 **Flush:** N/S, G, Hep/S **Sodium content:** 2 mmol/g **Displacement value:** Nil. Diluent takes displacement into account, e.g. 40 mg + 1 mL = 1 mL.	**Y-site compatible (but see Section A, 2.6):** aciclovir, dopamine, Hep/S, heparin, midazolam, morphine, linezolid, metronidazole, remifentanil. **Incompatible:** ciprofloxacin, cisatracurium, potassium chloride, propofol.
	(I) IV infusion (doses >250 mg)	Reconstitute as above then further dilute to a suitable volume with G, N/S or G/S. Fluid restriction: undiluted infusions have been given (anecdotal).	Min. 30 minutes.		
	IM (for doses up to 40 mg)	Reconstitute with diluent provided.			

- For abbreviations used in the Table, see Section A, 2.4.
  e.g. (C) IV = continuous intravenous infusion; (I) IV = intermittent intravenous infusion.
- Prepare a fresh infusion every 24 hours unless otherwise specified.
- Presume suitability as single-use only unless otherwise specified.
- Always check with additional reference sources regarding compatibility information – see Section A, 2.2.

Formulation	Method	Dilution	Rate	Comments	Compatibility
Methylthioninium chloride (methylene blue)					
Ampoule 1%, 5 mL	IV bolus (unlicensed) used in hypotension associated with sepsis and methaemaglobinaemia	Ready diluted.	Several minutes (as slow as possible).	**Acute events that may accompany administration:** Hypertension, monitor blood pressure. Rapid injection may produce additional methaemoglobinaemia. Extravasation may cause tissue damage; for management guidelines, see Section A, 7. **pH:** 3–4.5 **Flush:** N/S **Sodium content:** Nil **Other comments:** Manufacturer advises to administer through a sterile 0.45 μm filter.	
	(C) IV infusion (unlicensed) for methaemaglobinaemia.	Dilute in G/S to a convenient volume.			

Formulation	Method	Dilution	Rate	Comments	Compatibility
Metoclopramide					
Ampoule 10mg/2mL	IV bolus	May be diluted with N/S (usually 10–20mL).	1–2 minutes.	**Acute events that may accompany administration:** Dystonic reactions, particularly in children and young women. **pH:** 10mg/2mL = 3–5; 100mg/20mL = 5–7 **Flush:** N/S or G **Sodium content:** 10mg/2mL negligible, 100mg/20mL contains 2.74mmol Na^+.	**Compatibility in S/C syringe pump:** with diamorphine, see Section A, 8 for details **Y-site compatible (but see Section A, 2.6):** dexamethasone, heparin, hydrocortisone sodium succinate, insulin (soluble), magnesium sulphate, potassium chloride.
	IM	Ready diluted.			
	S/C bolus or (C) S/C infusion (widespread practice).	Ready diluted. May be further diluted with W or N/S.			

- For abbreviations used in the Table, see Section A, 2.4.
  e.g. (C) IV = continuous intravenous infusion; (I) IV = intermittent intravenous infusion.
- Prepare a fresh infusion every 24 hours unless otherwise specified.
- Presume suitability as single-use only unless otherwise specified.
- Always check with additional reference sources regarding compatibility information – see Section A, 2.2.

Formulation	Method	Dilution	Rate	Comments	Compatibility
Metoclopramide High Dose (Maxolon High Dose)					
Ampoule 100mg/20mL	(C) IV infusion (preferred method)	Loading dose 2–4mg/kg in 50–100mL N/S, G, G/S or H. Maintenance 3–5mg/kg in 500mL diluent.	Loading dose 15–30 minutes. Maintenance 8–12 hours.	Maxalon HD is not suitable for multidose use. Max. dose 10mg/kg in 24 hours.	
	(I) IV infusion	Up to 2mg/kg in a minimum of 50mL N/S, G, G/S or H.	Min. 15 minutes.		
Metoprolol					
Ampoule 5mg/5mL	IV bolus	May be diluted with N/S or G.	1–2mg/minute	**Acute events that may accompany administration:** Hypotension, bradycardia and cardiac arrhythmias. Monitor blood pressure and heart rate. **pH:** 5.5–7.5 **Flush:** N/S or G **Sodium content:** 0.8mmol/ampoule	
	(C) IV infusion (unlicensed ICU local practice) via syringe pump	May be diluted with N/S or G (e.g. 20mg in 50mL G).	Start at 0.04mg/kg per hour and titrate to response.		

162

Formulation	Method	Dilution	Rate	Comments	Compatibility
Metronidazole					
Infusion bag 500 mg/ 100 mL, Ampoule 100 mg/20 mL	(I) IV infusion	Infusion bag is ready diluted. Ampoules may be further diluted with N/S, G/S or G.	**Adults:** 25 mg/ minute (i.e. 500 mg over 20 minutes). **Children:** 20 minutes.	**pH:** 5–7 **Flush:** N/S, G or G/S **Sodium content:** 2.7 mmol/100 mg ampoule, 13.15 mmol/500 mg infusion.	Any one of amikacin, ceftazidime, cefotaxime and cefuroxime may be added to an infusion of metronidazole **Y-site compatible (but see Section A, 2.6):** aciclovir, aminophylline, amiodarone, amoxicillin, ciprofloxacin, clarithromycin, dopamine, fluconazole, foscarnet, gentamicin, heparin, magnesium sulphate, midazolam, morphine. piperacillin/tazobactam. **Incompatible:** G 10%, H, azlocillin, trimethoprim.

- For abbreviations used in the Table, see Section A, 2.4.
  e.g. (C) IV = continuous intravenous infusion; (I) IV = intermittent intravenous infusion.
- Prepare a fresh infusion every 24 hours unless otherwise specified.
- Presume suitability as single-use only unless otherwise specified.
- Always check with additional reference sources regarding compatibility information – see Section A, 2.2.

Formulation	Method	Dilution	Rate	Comments	Compatibility
Mexiletine					
Ampoule 250 mg/10 mL	IV bolus (loading dose)	Ready diluted.	25 mg/minute	**Acute events that may accompany administration:** Hypotension, monitor blood pressure. Sinus bradycardia, atrial fibrillation, atrioventricular dissociation and exacerbation of arrhythmias. Monitor **ECG**. **pH:** 5–6 **Flush:** N/S or G **Sodium content:** 0.3 mmol/10 mL	
	(C) IV infusion (may be used to load or provide maintenance dose).	See package insert for details. Dilute with 250–500 mL N/S or G.	See package insert for details		

Formulation	Method	Dilution	Rate	Comments	Compatibility
Midazolam					
Ampoule 10mg/2mL, 10mg/5mL	IV bolus	Ready diluted.	30 seconds minimum. Usually given over 2 minutes (approx. 2mg/minute) and repeated at intervals of at least 2 minutes.	**Acute events that may accompany administration:** Respiratory depression and arrest have occurred when doses are given too quickly. Should only be given when resuscitation facilities available. Paradoxical reactions such as aggression, hyperactivity and involuntary movements have been reported. This is associated with higher doses, rapid administration and among children and older patients. Extravasation may cause tissue damage; for management guidelines, see Section A, 7.	**Compatibility in S/C syringe pump:** with diamorphine, see Section A, 8 for details. **Y-site compatible (but see Section A, 2.6):** atracurium, dopamine, amiodarone, calcium gluconate, clindamycin, digoxin, dopamine, fluconazole, gentamicin, heparin, methylprednisolone sodium succinate, glyceryl trinitrate, sodium nitroprusside, vancomycin, vecuronium, potassium chloride, noradrenaline (norepinephrine), ciprofloxacin, insulin (soluble), metronidazole, fentanyl, morphine.

Midazolam cont'd on p. 166 overleaf

- For abbreviations used in the Table, see Section A, 2.4.
  e.g. (C) IV = continuous intravenous infusion; (I) IV = intermittent intravenous infusion.
- Prepare a fresh infusion every 24hours unless otherwise specified.
- Presume suitability as single-use only unless otherwise specified.
- Always check with additional reference sources regarding compatibility information – see Section A, 2.2.

Midazolam cont'd from p. 165

Formulation	Method	Dilution	Rate	Comments	Compatibility
	(C) IV infusion via syringe pump following initial loading dose over 5 minutes.	Dilute if required with N/S, G or G/S. May be administered undiluted. For neonates and children under 15kg dilute to a max. concentration 1mg/mL.		**pH**: 3 (approximately) **Flush:** N/S, G **Sodium content:** Negligible	**Incompatible:** amoxicillin, bumetanide, cefuroxime, co-amoxiclav, co-trimoxazole, dexamethasone, dobutamine, furosemide, foscarnet, imipenem, sodium bicarbonate, thiopental.
	(C) S/C infusion via syringe pump (unlicensed).	Dilute with W.			
	IM (painful).	Ready diluted.			

Formulation	Method	Dilution	Rate	Comments	Compatibility
Mivacurium					
Ampoule 10mg/5mL, 20mg/10mL	IV bolus	May be administered undiluted, or diluted with N/S, G or G/S to a concentration of 500 micrograms/1mL.	5–15 seconds, but see 'Other comments'.	**Acute events that may accompany administration:** Hypotension, monitor blood pressure. **pH:** 4.5 **Flush:** N/S **Sodium content:** Negligible **Other comments:** Doses up to 150 micrograms/kg may be given over 5–15 seconds, higher doses should be given over 30 seconds. Give IV bolus over 60 seconds to patients with cardiovascular disease, those with increased sensitivity to histamine (e.g. people with asthma) and those who may be unusually sensitive to falls in blood pressure. Histamine release may occur particularly with rapid injection.	**Y-site compatible (but see Section A, 2.6):** alfentanil, fentanyl, midazolam. **Incompatible:** alkaline agents, e.g. thiopental.
	(C) IV infusion	As above.	8–10 micrograms/kg per minute – adjusted according to patient response.		

- For abbreviations used in the Table, see Section A, 2.4.
  e.g. (C) IV = continuous intravenous infusion; (I) IV = intermittent intravenous infusion.
- Prepare a fresh infusion every 24 hours unless otherwise specified.
- Presume suitability as single-use only unless otherwise specified.
- Always check with additional reference sources regarding compatibility information – see Section A, 2.2.

167

Formulation	Method	Dilution	Rate	Comments	Compatibility
Morphine					
Ampoule 10 mg/1 mL, 30 mg/1 mL	IV bolus	May be diluted with N/S, G, G 10% or G/S.	3–5 minutes (2 mg/minute).	**Acute events that may accompany administration:** Severe respiratory depression, apnoea, hypotension, peripheral circulatory collapse, chest wall rigidity, cardiac arrest and anaphylactic shock. Monitor blood pressure, heart and respiratory rate. Extravasation may cause tissue damage; for management guidelines, see Section A, 7. **pH:** 3.0–6.0 **Flush:** N/S, G or G/S **Sodium content:** Negligible **Other comments:** Repeated S/C injections may cause local irritation, pain and induration.	**Compatibility in S/C syringe pump:** heparin, morphine 1 mg/1 mL and cyclizine < 2 mg/1 mL in N/S (local practice), metoclopramide. **Y-site compatible (but see Section A, 2.6):** aminophylline, atracurium, atropine, benzylpenicillin, bumetanide, cefotaxime, ceftazidime, cefuroxime, co-trimoxazole, dexamethasone, digoxin, dopamine, erythromycin, gentamicin, glycopyrronium, hydrocortisone sodium succinate, hyoscine butylbromide, insulin (soluble), ketamine, labetalol, lidocaine, magnesium sulphate, metoclopramide, metronidazole,

Formulation	Method	Dilution	Rate	Comments	Compatibility
	(C) IV infusion or (C) S/C infusion (unlicensed) via syringe pump.	Dilute in N/S or G usually to 1 mg/1 mL.			midazolam, ondansetron, pancuronium, potassium chloride, propofol (local practice), propranolol, suxamethonium, vancomycin, vecuronium. **Incompatible:** aciclovir, alkaline agents, aminophylline, flucloxacillin, furosemide, heparin, ketorolac, phenytoin, sodium bicarbonate, thiopental.
	IM or S/C. See 'Other comments'.	Ready diluted.			

- For abbreviations used in the Table, see Section A, 2.4.

  e.g. (C) IV = continuous intravenous infusion; (I) IV = intermittent intravenous infusion.

- Prepare a fresh infusion every 24 hours unless otherwise specified.
- Presume suitability as single-use only unless otherwise specified.
- Always check with additional reference sources regarding compatibility information – see Section A, 2.2.

Formulation	Method	Dilution	Rate	Comments	Compatibility
Mycophenolate Mofetil					
Vial 500 mg	(I) IV infusion	For a 1 g dose, reconstitute each 500 mg vial with 14 mL G. Add the contents of the two reconstituted vials to 140 mL of G. Final solution is 6 mg/mL.	120 minutes.	**Acute events that may accompany administration:** Hypersensitivity reactions have been reported. **pH:** 2.4–4.1 **Flush:** G **Other comments:** May be administered by either peripheral or central vein.	Do not mix or administer concurrently via the same catheter with other intravenous medicines or infusion admixtures. **Incompatible:** N/S.

Formulation	Method	Dilution	Rate	Comments	Compatibility
Naloxone					
Ampoule 40 micrograms/2mL, 400 micrograms/ 1mL	IV bolus	The 400 micrograms/ 1mL solution may be diluted with W or N/S immediately before use to a concentration of 20 micrograms/ 1mL.		**Acute events that may accompany administration:** Hypo- or hypertension, ventricular tachycardia and fibrillation. Precipitation of acute withdrawal syndrome. Extravasation may cause tissue damage; for management guidelines, see Section A. 7. **pH:** 3–4.5 **Flush:** N/S or G **Sodium content:** Negligible	**Y-site compatible (but see Section A, 2.6):** heparin, propofol. **Incompatible:** alkaline agents
	(C) or (I) IV infusion via syringe or volumetric infusion pump.	Dilute with G, G/S or N/S to 4 micrograms/ 1mL.	According to response.		
	IM or S/C	Ready diluted.			

- For abbreviations used in the Table, see Section A, 2.4.
  e.g. (C) IV = continuous intravenous infusion; (I) IV = intermittent intravenous infusion.
- Prepare a fresh infusion every 24hours unless otherwise specified.
- Presume suitability as single-use only unless otherwise specified.
- Always check with additional reference sources regarding compatibility information – see Section A, 2.2.

171

Formulation	Method	Dilution	Rate	Comments	Compatibility
Neostigmine					
Ampoule 2.5 mg/1 mL	IV bolus	May be diluted with W or N/S immediately before use.	Minimum 3–5 minutes. For reversal of non-depolarising neuromuscular blockade, over 1 minute.	**Acute events that may accompany administration:** Abdominal cramps, bradycardia, diarrhoea, salivation. Glycopyrronium or atropine should be given to prevent these muscarinic effects. **pH:** 4.5–6.5 **Flush:** N/S **Sodium content:** Negligible **Other comments:** Have atropine available to counteract possible cholinergic reactions.	**Y-site compatible (but see Section A, 2.6):** heparin, hydrocortisone sodium succinate, potassium chloride.
	IM or S/C	Ready diluted.			

Formulation	Method	Dilution	Rate	Comments	Compatibility
Nimodipine					
Vial 10mg/50mL (0.02%)	(I) IV infusion Must be administered centrally via a syringe pump connected to a three-way tap using the infusion line provided. Administer with a co-infusion of N/S or G running at a rate of 40mL/hour. See product information for full details	Ready diluted.	See package insert for details.	**Acute events that may accompany administration:** Hypotension, monitor blood pressure Tachycardia or bradycardia, monitor heart rate. Flushing can also occur. **pH:** 6–7.5 (undiluted infusion) **Flush:** N/S or G **Other comments:** Incompatible with PVC; use polyethylene or polypropylene apparatus provided. Protect infusion line and syringe from light. Contains alcohol.	Do not infuse with other medicines. Compatible with Dextran 40, human albumin 5%, mannitol.

- For abbreviations used in the Table, see Section A, 2.4.
  e.g. (C) IV = continuous intravenous infusion; (I) IV = intermittent intravenous infusion.
- Prepare a fresh infusion every 24 hours unless otherwise specified.
- Presume suitability as single-use only unless otherwise specified.
- Always check with additional reference sources regarding compatibility information – see Section A, 2.2.

Formulation	Method	Dilution	Rate	Comments	Compatibility
Noradrenaline (norepinephrine) acid tartrate					
Ampoule 4 mg/2 mL (equivalent to 2 mg/2 mL noradrenaline base)	(C) or (I) IV infusion into a central line via syringe pump.	Standard dilution: 2, 4, 8 or 16 mg noradrenaline base/50 mL in G/S or G. Infuse via a central line (local practice). Higher or lower concentrations may be prepared if necessary. Undiluted solutions have been used (anecdotal).	Adjust rate according to response.	**Acute events that may accompany administration:** Avoid peripheral administration because extravasation can produce local vasoconstriction leading to severe tissue hypoxia and ischaemia; for management guidelines, see Section A. 7. Noradrenaline infusions should only be used in areas where appropriate cardiovascular monitoring is available (ITU, HDU, etc.). **pH:** 3–4.5 (undiluted) **Do not flush:** Replace giving set **Other comments:** pH of diluent must be ≤ 6. Loss of potency occurs if diluent is N/S. Discard infusion if brown colour develops.	**Y-site compatible (but see Section A, 2.6):** adrenaline (epinephrine), amiodarone, calcium salts, dobutamine, dopamine, gentamicin, heparin, insulin (soluble), isoprenaline, lidocaine, magnesium sulphate, potassium chloride. **Incompatibe:** alkaline solutions, aminophylline, chlorphenamine, furosemide, phenytoin, sodium bicarbonate, thiopental.

Formulation	Method	Dilution	Rate	Comments	Compatibility
Octreotide					
Ampoule 50 micrograms/1mL, 100 micrograms/1ml, 500 micrograms/ 1mL	S/C (preferred method).	Dilution is not required.		**Acute events that may accompany administration:** Bradycardia, hypotension, facial flushing, hyperglycaemia and rarely hypoglycaemia. Monitor cardiac rhythms, **ECG**, blood glucose, blood pressure and heart rate with IV doses. Extravasation may cause tissue damage; for management guidelines, see Section A, 7. Rapid administration of the IV bolus may produce stinging at the injection site and a brief drop in heart rate. **pH:** 3.9–4.5 **Flush:** N/S **Sodium content:** Negligible **Other comments:** To reduce local discomfort, let solution reach room temperature before injection. When administered subcutaneously, smaller volumes cause less discomfort. Diluted solutions should be discarded after 24 hours (local practice).	**Y-site compatible (but see Section A, 2.6):** heparin. **Incompatible:** cyclizine, insulin (soluble), steroids.
	IV bolus	Dilute dose with N/S to a ratio of not less than 1:1 and not more than 1:9 by volume. Use immediately.	3–5 minutes.		
	(C) S/C infusion (unlicensed) via syringe pump.	Dilute dose to a suitable volume with N/S (local practice).			
	(I) or (C) IV infusion (unlicensed) via syringe pump.	Dilute dose to 50mL with N/S, i.e. to a ratio of not less than 1:1 and not more than 1:9 volume.	10–24 hours.		

- For abbreviations used in the Table, see Section A, 2.4.
- e.g. (C) IV = continuous intravenous infusion; (I) IV = intermittent intravenous infusion.
- Prepare a fresh infusion every 24 hours unless otherwise specified.
- Presume suitability as single-use only unless otherwise specified.
- Always check with additional reference sources regarding compatibility information – see Section A, 2.2.

175

Formulation	Method	Dilution	Rate	Comments	Compatibility
Omeprazole					
Vial 40mg for infusion, Vial 40mg for injection	(I) IV infusion	Reconstitute each 40mg vial 'for infusion' with 5mL N/S or G. Dilute in 100mL N/S or G.	20–30 minutes.	**Acute events that may accompany administration:** Visual impairment reported with high dose injection. Extravasation may cause tissue damage; for management guidelines, see Section A, 7. **pH:** infusion 9–10. IV injection 8.8–9.2 **Flush:** N/S, G **Sodium content:** Negligible **Other comments:** Revert to oral therapy as soon as possible. Use infusion in N/S within 12 hours, or 3 hours if in G. Use reconstituted solution for bolus injection within 3 hours.	Do not infuse with other medicines or infusion fluids.
	IV bolus	Reconstitute each 40mg vial for injection with the solvent provided.	Over 5 minutes.		
	(C) IV infusion	Reconstitute each 40mg vial 'for infusion' with 5mL N/S or G. Dilute, e.g. 200mg in 50mL (anecdotal).	8mg/hour		

Formulation	Method	Dilution	Rate	Comments	Compatibility
Ondansetron					
Ampoule 4mg/2mL, 8mg/4mL	IV bolus	May be diluted with N/S or G.	3–5 minutes.	**Acute events that may accompany administration:** Extravasation may cause tissue damage; for management guidelines, see Section A, 7. Hypersensitivity reactions around the injection site, sometimes extending along the medicine administration line. **pH:** 3.3–4.0 **Flush:** N/S **Sodium content:** Negligible	**Incompatible:** aciclovir, amphotericin, amsacrine, alkaline agents, fluconazole, ganciclovir, lorazepam, meropenem, sodium bicarbonate.
	(C) IV infusion	Dilute in a suitable volume of N/S or G.	1 mg/hour		
	(I) IV infusion	Dilute in 50–100mL N/S or G.	15 minutes.		
	IM (maximum volume at one site 2mL).	Ready diluted.			
	(C) S/C infusion (local practice).	Dilute to a suitable volume with W or N/S.			

- For abbreviations used in the Table, see Section A, 2.4.
  e.g. (C) IV = continuous intravenous infusion; (I) IV = intermittent intravenous infusion.
- Prepare a fresh infusion every 24hours unless otherwise specified.
- Presume suitability as single-use only unless otherwise specified.
- Always check with additional reference sources regarding compatibility information – see Section A, 2.2.

Formulation	Method	Dilution	Rate	Comments	Compatibility
Oxytocin					
Ampoule 5 units/1 mL, 10 units/1 mL	(C) IV infusion via volumetric infusion pump.	**Induction/ enhancement of labour:** dilute 10 units in 500 mL N/S or H (local practice). **Incomplete, inevitable or missed abortion:** 5 units by slow IV bolus followed by infusion of 40 units/500 mL H if necessary. **Treatment of postpartum uterine haemorrhage (PPH):** 5 units by slow IV bolus followed by an infusion of 5–20 units in 500 mL H if necessary.	Consult specialist information.	**Acute events that may accompany administration:** Uterine spasm, uterine hyperstimulation, nausea, vomiting and arrhythmias. Monitor maternal and foetal heart rate and blood pressure. Rapid infusion may cause an acute short-lasting hypotension accompanied by flushing and reflex tachycardia. Extravasation may cause tissue damage; for management guidelines, see Section A, 7. **pH:** 3.7–4.3 **Flush:** N/S, G **Other comments:** When high doses are administered over long periods, an electrolyte-containing diluent (not G) must be used. The volume of infused fluid should be kept low and fluid intake by mouth restricted, to prevent water intoxication and associated hyponatraemia. Close monitoring of patient's fluid and electrolyte status essential.	**Compatible fluids:** N/S, G, H, Ringer's. **Y-site compatible (but see Section A, 2.6):** Hep/S, potassium chloride. **Incompatible:** solutions containing sodium metabisulphite.

Formulation	Method	Dilution	Rate	Comments	Compatibility
	IV bolus	**Prevention of PPH:** 5 units, ready diluted.	2–3 minutes.		
	IM (unlicensed)	**PPH prophylaxis:** ready diluted.			

- For abbreviations used in the Table, see Section A, 2.4.
  e.g. (C) IV = continuous intravenous infusion; (I) IV = intermittent intravenous infusion.
- Prepare a fresh infusion every 24 hours unless otherwise specified.
- Presume suitability as single-use only unless otherwise specified.
- Always check with additional reference sources regarding compatibility information – see Section A, 2.2.

179

Formulation	Method	Dilution	Rate	Comments	Compatibility
Pabrinex IVHP (high potency)					
Ampoule no. 1 contains: pyridoxine 50 mg, riboflavine 4 mg and thiamine 250 mg in 5 mL. Ampoule no. 2 contains: ascorbic acid 500 mg, glucose 1 g and nicotinamide 160 mg in 5 mL	(I) IV infusion (preferred method).	Draw the contents of ampoules no. 1 and no. 2 (one pair of ampoules) into one syringe and mix. Add to 50–100 mL N/S or G.	15–30 minutes.	**Acute events that may accompany administration:** Anaphylaxis. Mild allergic reactions such as sneezing or mild asthma are warning signs that further injections may give rise to anaphylactic shock. Facilities for treating anaphylaxis must be available. **pH:** 4.9 when mixed **Flush:** N/S, G **Sodium content:** 2.95 mmol per pair of ampoules. **Other comments:** In thiamine deficiency avoid parenteral glucose as it may worsen symptoms and increase thiamine requirements.	**Compatible:** H **Incompatible:** amphotericin, calcium gluconate, chloramphenicol, erythromycin, tetracyclines.
	IV bolus	Draw the contents of each pair of ampoules into one syringe and mix.	10 minutes.		

180

Formulation	Method	Dilution	Rate	Comments	Compatibility
Pamidronate disodium					
Vial 15mg, 30mg, 90mg. Solution 15mg in 5mL, 30mg in 10mL, 60mg in 10mL, 90mg in 10mL	(I) IV infusion preferably into a large vein.	Reconstitute each 15mg with 5mL W. Further dilute with N/S, G or G/S. The final concentration should not exceed 60mg/250mL.	Maximum rate 60mg/hour. However, in renal impairment the recommended rate is 20mg/hour.	**Acute events that may accompany administration:** Hyper-or hypotension, monitor blood pressure. Dizziness or sleepiness – patients should be warned against driving after treatment. Fever and flu-like symptoms, treat with paracetamol. Local reactions such as pain, redness, induration, phlebitis and thrombophlebitis. **pH:** 6–7 **Flush:** N/S **Sodium content:** Negligible	**Incompatible:** calcium-containing solutions.

- For abbreviations used in the Table, see Section A, 2.4.
  e.g. (C) IV = continuous intravenous infusion; (I) IV = intermittent intravenous infusion.
- Prepare a fresh infusion every 24 hours unless otherwise specified.
- Presume suitability as single-use only unless otherwise specified.
- Always check with additional reference sources regarding compatibility information – see Section A, 2.2.

Formulation	Method	Dilution	Rate	Comments	Compatibility
Pancuronium					
Ampoule 4 mg/2 mL	IV bolus	May be diluted with G or N/S.	30 seconds.	**Acute events that may accompany administration:** Tachycardia and rise in arterial pressure and cardiac output. Monitor heart rate and blood pressure. Extravasation may cause tissue damage; for management guidelines, see Section A, 7. **pH:** 3.8–4.2 **Flush:** N/S or G **Sodium content:** 0.28 mmol/2 mL **Other comments:** Do not add medicines to the same syringe as a fall in pH may cause precipitation.	**Y-site compatible (but see Section A, 2.6):** alfentanil, aminophylline, co-trimoxazole, dobutamine, Dextran 40, fentanyl, gentamicin, heparin, hydrocortisone sodium succinate, isoprenaline, midazolam, morphine, propofol, sodium nitroprusside. **Incompatible:** Phenobarbital.
	(I) or (C) IV infusion via a syringe pump (continuous infusion unlicensed).	May be diluted with G or N/S.	Dependent on patient response.		
	IM (unlicensed).	Ready diluted.			

Formulation	Method	Dilution	Rate	Comments	Compatibility
Papaveretum					
Ampoule 15.4mg/1mL	IM or S/C (preferred method); see 'Other comments'.	Ready diluted.		**Acute events that may accompany administration:** Respiratory depression, hypotension, sedation, anaphylaxis, nausea and vomiting. Monitor blood pressure, heart rate, respiratory rate, sedation score. **pH:** 2.5–4 **Flush:** N/S **Sodium content:** Negligible **Other comments:** IM injection is preferred to S/C as it is less irritant. IM injections should be injected into large muscle mass to avoid nerve trunks.	
	(C) IV infusion via syringe pump (unlicensed).	Dilute with N/S or G.			
	IV bolus	Dilute with W, N/S or G.	2–3 minutes.		

- For abbreviations used in the Table, see Section A, 2.4.
  e.g. (C) IV = continuous intravenous infusion; (I) IV = intermittent intravenous infusion.
- Prepare a fresh infusion every 24 hours unless otherwise specified.
- Presume suitability as single-use only unless otherwise specified.
- Always check with additional reference sources regarding compatibility information – see Section A, 2.2.

183

Formulation	Method	Dilution	Rate	Comments	Compatibility
Paracetamol					
Vial 500mg in 50mL, 1g in 100mL	(I) IV infusion	Ready diluted.	15 minutes.	**Acute events that may accompany administration:** Acute infusion reactions – monitor patient; very rarely hypersensitivity may occur. **Flush:** N/S **Sodium content:** Not greater than 0.17 mmol/100 mL vial. **Displacement:** N/A. **pH:** 5.5 **Other comments:** IV paracetamol is the same dose as standard oral paracetamol and rectal paracetamol.	Do not infuse with other medicines.

Formulation	Method	Dilution	Rate	Comments	Compatibility
Pentamidine					
Vial 300mg	(I) IV infusion with patient supine.	Reconstitute with 3–5mL W. Withdraw the appropriate dose and dilute with 50–250mL N/S or G.	Minimum 1 hour. For prehydration see 'Other comments'.	**Acute events that may accompany administration:** May cause sudden, severe hypotension; to reduce risk – keep patient supine. Baseline blood pressure should be established before infusion and monitored every 15 minutes during and 1 hour post-infusion. Local reactions can occur with varying severity. **pH:** 4.5–6.5 (5% solution) **Flush:** N/S or G **Sodium content:** Nil **Displacement:** 0.15mL/300mg Add 4.85mL W to 300mg vial to give a concentration of 60mg/1mL. **Other comments:** Consider pre-hydration to reduce renal toxicity in susceptible patients with 500mL–1L N/S, depending on fluid tolerance. Caution in handling. Pentamidine is toxic. Adequate protection required during handling and administration. Consult product literature. IM injections should be deep and preferably given in the buttock.	Do not infuse with other medicines.
	IM (not recommended in HIV).	Reconstitute with 3mL W.			

- For abbreviations used in the Table, see Section A, 2.4.
  e.g. (C) IV = continuous intravenous infusion; (I) IV = intermittent intravenous infusion.
- Prepare a fresh infusion every 24hours unless otherwise specified.
- Presume suitability as single-use only unless otherwise specified.
- Always check with additional reference sources regarding compatibility information – see Section A, 2.2.

Formulation	Method	Dilution	Rate	Comments	Compatibility
Pethidine					
Ampoule 50mg/1mL, 100mg/2mL	IV bolus	May be diluted with W, N/S or G to a concentration of 10mg/1mL.	2–3 minutes.	**Acute events that may accompany administration:** Respiratory depression, hypotension, sedation, anaphylaxis, nausea and vomiting. Monitor blood pressure, heart rate, respiratory rate, sedation score. **pH:** 4.5–6 **Flush:** N/S or G **Sodium content:** Nil **Other comments:** The IM route is preferred to S/C for repeated injections. This is because of occurrence of irritation and induration at the S/C injection site.	**Y-site compatible (but see Section A, 2.6):** amphotericin, bumetanide, hyoscine butylbromide, glycopyrronium, insulin (soluble), labetalol, potassium chloride, propranolol. **Incompatible:** aciclovir, aminophylline, ephedrine, heparin, hydrocortisone sodium succinate, imipenem, ketorolac, methylprednisolone, phenobarbital, phenytoin, sodium bicarbonate, thiopental.
	(C) IV infusion (unlicensed) via volumetric infusion or syringe pump.	Dilute with N/S, G or H.			
	IM into large muscle mass. See 'Other comments'.	Ready diluted.			
	S/C. See 'Other comments'.	Ready diluted.			

Formulation	Method	Dilution	Rate	Comments	Compatibility
Phenobarbital (phenobarbitone)					
Ampoule 15 mg/1 mL, 30 mg/1 mL, 60 mg/1 mL, 200 mg/1 mL	IV bolus	Dilute to 10 times its own volume with **W** immediately before use.	Maximum rate in children is 1 mg/kg per min. Rate in adults should not exceed 100 mg/minute.	**Acute events that may accompany administration:** Sedation, hypotension, tachycardia, respiratory depression. Monitor sedation score, respiratory rate, heart rate and blood pressure. Extravasation may cause tissue damage; for management guidelines, see Section A, 7. **pH:** 9–10.5 **Flush:** N/S **Sodium content per ampoule:** Negligible	**Incompatible:** acidic solutions, including, chlorpromazine, ephedrine, G, pethidine, vancomycin.
	(I) IV infusion via syringe pump.	As above.			
	IM	May dilute with **W** to a suitable volume.			

- For abbreviations used in the Table, see Section A, 2.4.
  e.g. (C) IV = continuous intravenous infusion; (I) IV = intermittent intravenous infusion.
- Prepare a fresh infusion every 24 hours unless otherwise specified.
- Presume suitability as single-use only unless otherwise specified.
- Always check with additional reference sources regarding compatibility information – see Section A, 2.2.

187

Formulation	Method	Dilution	Rate	Comments	Compatibility
Phenoxybenzamine					
Ampoule 100 mg/2 mL	(I) IV infusion via volumetric infusion pump. Infuse into a large vein.	Dilute with 200–500 mL N/S.	Minimum 2 hours.	**Acute events that may accompany administration:** Hypotension, monitor blood pressure every few minutes. Extravasation may cause tissue damage; for management guidelines. see Section A, 7. **pH:** 2.5–3.1 **Flush:** N/S **Other comments:** Discard infusion 4 hours after dilution. Avoid hand contamination due to the risk of contact sensitisation.	
Phentolamine mesilate					
Ampoule 10 mg/1 mL	IV bolus	Ready diluted.	Rapidly.	**Acute events that may accompany administration:** Tachycardia, arrhythmias and hypotension; monitor **ECG** and blood pressure. Presence of sulphites in preparation (especially in patients with asthma) may lead to hypersensitivity reactions. **Flush:** N/S, G or G/S **pH:** 3–5	
	IM	Ready diluted.			

Formulation	Method	Dilution	Rate	Comments	Compatibility
Phenylephrine					
Ampoule 10 mg/1 mL (10000 micrograms/ 1 mL)	IV bolus	Dilute 1 mg (1000 micrograms) with 1 mL W.	100–500 micrograms over 3–5 minutes.	**Acute events that may accompany administration:** Respiratory distress, hypertension, headache, tremor, bradycardia, palpitations and vomiting. Can cause severe peripheral and visceral vasoconstriction and volume depletion. Extravasation may cause local tissue necrosis; for management guidelines, see Section A, 7. Monitor blood pressure and heart rate during IV infusions and regularly post-IM or S/C injections. Ensure that patient is not volume depleted before infusion. **pH:** 4.5–6.5 **Flush:** N/S or G	**Y-site compatible (but see Section A, 2.6):** aminophylline, amiodarone, dobutamine, heparin, lidocaine. **Incompatible:** phenytoin, alkaline solutions.
	(I) IV infusion via volumetric infusion pump.	Add 10 mg to 500 mL N/S or G.	Up to 180 micrograms/ minute reduced according to response to 30–60 micrograms/ minute.		
	IM or S/C	Ready diluted.	Maximum single dose 5 mg.		

- For abbreviations used in the Table, see Section A, 2.4.
  e.g. (C) IV = continuous intravenous infusion; (I) IV = intermittent intravenous infusion.
- Prepare a fresh infusion every 24 hours unless otherwise specified.
- Presume suitability as single-use only unless otherwise specified.
- Always check with additional reference sources regarding compatibility information – see Section A, 2.2.

189

Formulation	Method	Dilution	Rate	Comments	Compatibility
Phenytoin sodium					
Ampoule 250 mg/5 mL	IV bolus (preferred method). Inject via a large needle into a large vein.	Unless essential do not dilute as precipitation may occur.	**Adults:** max rate 50 mg/minute **Neonates:** 1–3 mg/kg per minute.	**Acute events that may accompany administration:** Arrhythmias: **ECG** monitoring recommended. Hypotension: monitor blood pressure. Respiratory and CNS depression (particularly if injected too rapidly). Extravasation may cause tissue damage; for management guidelines, see Section A, 7. To avoid local venous irritation flush line with N/S before and after each infusion or injection. **pH:** 12 **Flush:** N/S **Sodium content:** 0.91 mmol/250 mg **Other comments:** Plasma level monitoring is required. Complete administration within 1 hour of preparation.	**Y-site compatible (but see Section A, 2.6):** foscarnet, fluconazole. **Incompatible:** ciprofloxacin, clarithromycin, heparin sodium, insulin (soluble), lidocaine, morphine, pethidine, potassium chloride, propofol.
	(I) IV infusion via syringe or volumetric infusion pump. Inject via a large needle into a large vein.	Dilute in 50–100 mL N/S to a final concentration not exceeding 10 mg/1 mL. Stable for 1 hour. Use an in-line 0.2–0.50 μm filter. Do not use if solution is hazy or contains precipitate.	See above.		

Formulation	Method	Dilution	Rate	Comments	Compatibility
Phosphates neutral					
Polyfusor 50mmol/500mL	(I) IV infusion	Ready diluted.	Usual maximum rate 9mmol phosphate over 12 hours (7.5mL/hour). Faster rates are used on ITU, e.g. up to 50mmol/24 hours (local practice).	**Acute events that may accompany administration:** Oedema and hypotension: monitor blood pressure. Doses exceeding 9mmol/12 hours may cause hypocalcaemia and metastatic calcification; monitor calcium, phosphate, potassium, other electrolytes and renal function. **pH:** 7–7.8 **Flush:** N/S	

- For abbreviations used in the Table, see Section A, 2.4.
  e.g. (C) IV = continuous intravenous infusion; (I) IV = intermittent intravenous infusion.
- Prepare a fresh infusion every 24 hours unless otherwise specified.
- Presume suitability as single-use only unless otherwise specified.
- Always check with additional reference sources regarding compatibility information – see Section A, 2.2.

Formulation	Method	Dilution	Rate	Comments	Compatibility
Phytomenadione (Konakion MM)					
Ampoule 10mg/1mL (1mL adult), Ampoule 10mg/1mL (0.2mL paediatric)	IV bolus	Ready diluted.	3–5 minutes.	**Acute events that may accompany administration:** Possible anaphylactoid reactions. **pH:** 5.5–6.3 **Flush:** G, N/S **Other comments:** The manufacturer recommends the use of non-siliconised syringes, e.g. BBraun. Do not further dilute the 0.2mL ampoule.	
	(I) IV infusion	**Adults:** add to 55mL G before administration.	15–30 minutes.		

192

Formulation	Method	Dilution	Rate	Comments	Compatibility
Piperacillin and tazobactam					
Vial 2.25 g containing piperacillin 2 g and tazobactam 250 mg. Vial 4.5 g containing piperacillin 4 g and tazobactam 500 mg	IV bolus	Reconstitute the 2.25 g vial with 10 mL W or N/S, and the 4.5 g vial with 20 mL of W or N/S.	3–5 minutes.	**Acute events that may accompany administration:** Thrombophlebitis; anaphylaxis. **pH:** 4.5–7 **Flush:** N/S **Sodium content:** 4.5 mmol/2.25 g, 9 mmol/4.5 g **Displacement:** 1.6 mL/2.25 g Add 8.4 mL diluent to 2.25 g vial to give a concentration of 225 mg/1 mL.	**Y-site compatible (but see Section A, 2.6):** folinic acid, potassium chloride. **Incompatible:** amphotericin, aminoglycosides, sodium bicarbonate.
	(I) IV infusion	Reconstitute as above, then dilute to a convenient volume with N/S, G or G/S.	20–30 minutes.		

- For abbreviations used in the Table, see Section A, 2.4.
- e.g. (C) IV = continuous intravenous infusion; (I) IV = intermittent intravenous infusion.
- Prepare a fresh infusion every 24 hours unless otherwise specified.
- Presume suitability as single-use only unless otherwise specified.
- Always check with additional reference sources regarding compatibility information – see Section A, 2.2.

193

Formulation	Method	Dilution	Rate	Comments	Compatibility
Potassium canrenoate (unlicensed)					
Ampoule 200mg/10mL	IV bolus preferably not into a small vein	Ready diluted.	Max. rate 100mg/minute	**Acute events that may accompany administration:** If the undiluted solution is injected too quickly pain and irritation at the injection site may occur. Transient confusion may occur during high dose therapy (>1g daily). Extravasation may cause tissue damage; for management guidelines, see Section A, 7. **pH:** 10.7–11.2 **Flush:** N/S or G **Other comments:** Use infusion within 12 hours.	Do not infuse with other medicines.
	(I) IV infusion	Dilute to 250mL with N/S or G (G is preferred if ascites present).	90 minutes.		

Formulation	Method	Dilution	Rate	Comments	Compatibility
Potassium chloride					
Infusion bag 10mmol in 500mL N/S, 20mmol in 500mL N/S, 20mmol in 1L N/S, 40mmol in 1L N/S, 10mmol in 500mL G, 20mmol in 1L G, 20mmol in 500mL G, 40mmol in 1L G, 10mmol in 500mL G/S, 20mmol in 1L G/S, 20mmol in 500mL G/S, 40mmol in 1L G/S,	(C) IV infusion into a peripheral line via a volumetric infusion pump.	Maximum concentration 40mmol/L. Use ready-prepared infusion bags containing potassium 20mmol/L and 40mmol/L in N/S, G or G/S. MIX THOROUGH-LY.	**Adults:** usual suggested max. rate 10mmol potassium/hour **Children:** usual max. rate 0.2mmol potassium/kg per hour up to a maximum of 10mmol/hour Note: faster rates have been used in severe depletion with **ECG** monitoring, e.g. 20mmol/hour (anecdotal)	**Acute events that may accompany administration: ECG** monitoring should be used when the rate exceeds 20mmol/hour. Administration of 40mmol over a period of less than 1 hour poses a serious risk of asystole. Pain or phlebitis may occur during peripheral administration of solutions containing more than 30mmol/L of potassium. Extravasation may cause tissue damage; for management guidelines, see Section A, 7. **pH:** 3.5–6.5 **Flush:** N/S	**Y-site compatible (but see Section A, 2.6):** aciclovir, adrenaline (epinephrine), amiodarone, aminophylline, atracurium, atropine, calcium gluconate, ciprofloxacin, clarithromycin, clindamycin, digoxin, dobutamine, dopamine, fentanyl, flucloxacillin, fluconazole, furosemide, heparin, hydralazine, hydrocortisone sodium succinate, insulin (soluble), labetalol, lidocaine, lorazepam, magnesium sulphate, midazolam, noradrenaline (norepinephrine),

Potassium chloride cont'd on p. 196 overleaf

- For abbreviations used in the Table, see Section A, 2.4.
  e.g. (C) IV = continuous intravenous infusion; (I) IV = intermittent intravenous infusion.
- Prepare a fresh infusion every 24 hours unless otherwise specified.
- Presume suitability as single-use only unless otherwise specified.
- Always check with additional reference sources regarding compatibility information – see Section A, 2.2.

195

Formulation	Method	Dilution	Rate	Comments	Compatibility
Ampoule 1.5 g/10 mL (20 mmol), 20 mmol in 100 mL N/S (special), 40 mmol in 100 mL N/S (special), 60 mmol in 1000 mL N/S (special), 80 mmol in 1000 mL N/S (special), Other specials are available.	(C) or (I) IV infusion into a central line via a syringe or volumetric infusion pump.	Dilute to required concentration with N/S, G or G/S and MIX THOROUGH-TY. Concentrations >40 mmol/L are only given at UCLH on ICU, coronary care, neonatal, haematology and oncology wards. ICU local practice: 40 mmol in 50 mL G centrally only.	See above.	The NPSA's alert now requires Trusts to: • restrict potassium chloride concentrate to pharmacy departments and critical care areas. • remove potassium chloride concentrate from wards. • use commercially prepared diluted potassium solution where possible. • store potassium chloride concentrate in a separate locked cupboard away from other common diluents such as sodium chloride solution. • ensure that preparation and administration of the medicine are checked by a second practitioner. • ensure appropriate training of all staff.	ondansetron, oxytocin, pethidine, piperacillin/tazobactam, procainamide, propofol, propranolol, ranitidine, sodium bicarbonate, suxamethonium. **Incompatible:** amphotericin, methylprednisolone sodium succinate, phenytoin.

Formulation	Method	Dilution	Rate	Comments	Compatibility
Procainamide					
Vial 1g/10mL	IV bolus (for acute control of tachyarrhy-thmia).	May be diluted with G.	Max. rate 50mg/minute	**Acute events that may accompany administration:** Hypotension and myocardial toxicity, monitor blood pressure and **ECG.** Hypersensitivity reactions. **pH:** 4.5–5.5 **Flush:** G or N/S, Hep/S **Other comments:** Solution initially colourless but may turn slightly yellow on standing.	**Y-site compatible (but see Section A, 2.6):** amiodarone, dobutamine, heparin, lidocaine, potassium chloride. **Incompatible:** esmolol, milrinone, phenytoin.
	(I) and then (C) IV infusion via volumetric infusion pump (for suppression of chronic arrhythmias).	Dilute to 2–4mg/1mL with G.	Adult loading dose: infuse over 25–30 minutes then infuse maintenance dose at 2–6mg/minute		

- For abbreviations used in the Table, see Section A, 2.4.
- e.g. (C) IV = continuous intravenous infusion; (I) IV = intermittent intravenous infusion.
- Prepare a fresh infusion every 24 hours unless otherwise specified.
- Presume suitability as single-use only unless otherwise specified.
- Always check with additional reference sources regarding compatibility information – see Section A, 2.2.

Formulation	Method	Dilution	Rate	Comments	Compatibility
Prochlorperazine					
Ampoule 12.5 mg/1 mL	IV bolus (unlicensed)	Dilute 1 part with 9 parts N/S by volume before administration.	Max. rate 5 mg/ minute (max. dose 10 mg by this route).	**Acute events that may accompany administration:** Venospasm and postural hypotension; monitor blood pressure and heart rate. Rapid administration may irritate veins. Extravasation may cause tissue damage; for management guidelines, see Section A, 7. **pH:** 5.5–6.6 **Flush:** N/S **Sodium content:** Negligible	Do not infuse with other medicines.
	Deep IM	Ready diluted.			

Formulation	Method	Dilution	Rate	Comments	Compatibility
Procyclidine					
Ampoule 10 mg/2 mL	IV bolus	Ready diluted.		**Flush:** N/S	
	IM	Ready diluted.			
Promethazine					
Ampoule 25 mg/1 mL	Deep IM (preferred method)	Ready diluted.		**Acute events that may accompany administration:** Pain at injection site. Hypersensitivity reactions, hypotension, monitor blood pressure. Extravasation may cause tissue damage; for management guidelines, see Section A, 7. **pH:** 5–6 **Flush:** N/S, G	**Y-site compatible (but see Section A, 2.6):** G, N/S **Incompatible:** alkaline agents, ketorolac, heparin sodium.
	IV bolus	Dilute 1 part with 9 parts W before administration.	Give slowly. Max. rate 25 mg/minute		

- For abbreviations used in the Table, see Section A, 2.4.
  e.g. (C) IV = continuous intravenous infusion; (I) IV = intermittent intravenous infusion.
- Prepare a fresh infusion every 24 hours unless otherwise specified.
- Presume suitability as single-use only unless otherwise specified.
- Always check with additional reference sources regarding compatibility information – see Section A, 2.2.

199

Formulation	Method	Dilution	Rate	Comments	Compatibility
Propofol					
Ampoule 200mg/20mL, Vial 500mg/50mL, 1000mg/100mL	IV bolus	Ready diluted. May be administered into a Y-site (close to the injection site) of infusions of N/S, G or G/S.	**Adults:** usual dose 1.5–2.5mg/kg given in 20–40mg increments every 10 seconds	**Acute events that may accompany administration:** Hypotension, monitor airway obstruction and oxygen desaturation. **pH:** 7–7.1 **Flush:** N/S **Other comments:** Discard any unused diluted infusion after 6 hours. Should not be given via a microbiological filter. Can be used undiluted from plastic containers. There should be no significant loss of medicine unless left stagnant. If diluted in PVC, bag should be full and dilution prepared by withdrawing fluid and replacing with equal volume of propofol.	**Y-site compatible (but see Section A, 2.6):** alfentanil, atropine, morphine (local practice), pancuronium, suxamethonium, vecuronium. **Incompatible:** atracurium, mivacurium.
	(C) IV infusion via syringe or volumetric infusion pump.	Dependent on brand; see package insert.	Dependent on indication; see package insert.		

Formulation	Method	Dilution	Rate	Comments	Compatibility
Propranolol					
Ampoule 1 mg/1 mL	IV bolus	May be diluted with N/S, G/S or G.	**Adults:** max. rate 1 mg/minute	**Acute events that may accompany administration:** Bradycardia; monitor **ECG**. Extravasation may cause tissue damage; for management guidelines, see Section A, 7. **pH:** 3 **Flush:** N/S **Sodium content:** Nil	**Y-site compatible (but see Section A, 2.6):** heparin, morphine, pethidine, potassium chloride. **Incompatible:** decomposes rapidly at alkaline pH.
Prostacyclin					
	See Epoprostenol				
Prostaglandin E₁					
	See Alprostadil				

- For abbreviations used in the Table, see Section A, 2.4.
  e.g. (C) IV = continuous intravenous infusion; (I) IV = intermittent intravenous infusion.
- Prepare a fresh infusion every 24 hours unless otherwise specified.
- Presume suitability as single-use only unless otherwise specified.
- Always check with additional reference sources regarding compatibility information – see Section A, 2.2.

Formulation	Method	Dilution	Rate	Comments	Compatibility
Protamine sulphate					
Ampoule 50 mg/5 mL, 100 mg/10 mL	IV bolus via a peripheral vein.	May be diluted with N/S or G.	10 minutes (max. rate 5 mg/minute).	**Acute events that may accompany administration:** Monitor APTT coagulation tests. Rapid administration may cause hypotension, bradycardia and dyspnoea. Hypersensitivity reactions reported. Extravasation may cause tissue damage; for management guidelines, see Section A, 7. **pH:** 2.5–3.5 **Flush:** N/S **Sodium content:** 0.77 mmol/5 mL	
Protirelin					
Ampoule 200 mg/2 mL	IV bolus (diagnostic test)	Ready diluted.	30 seconds.	**Acute events that may accompany administration:** Hypertension, tachycardia and bronchospasm. The patient should be lying down during administration to reduce hypotension. Monitor blood pressure and heart rate. **pH:** 4.5–6.5 **Flush:** N/S	

Formulation	Method	Dilution	Rate	Comments	Compatibility
Quinine dihydrochloride					
Ampoule 300 mg/1 mL, 600 mg/2 mL	(I) IV infusion via volumetric infusion pump.	Add required dose to 250 mL preferably in N/S (otherwise G or G 10%). Normal maximum concentration is 2.4 mg/1 mL (local practice).	4 hours.	**Acute events that may accompany administration:** Hypoglycaemia; monitor blood glucose levels. Monitor for signs of cardiotoxicity. Cinchonism including tinnitis, headache, nausea, abdominal pain and visual disturbances. Fever and hypersensitivity such as flushing of skin and intense pruritis. Extravasation may cause tissue damage; for management guidelines, see Section A, 7. **pH:** 1.5–3 **Flush:** N/S or G	
	IM into anterior thigh (unlicensed).	Dilute in N/S to 60 mg/1 mL and give half dose into each thigh (local practice).			

- For abbreviations used in the Table, see Section A, 2.4.
  e.g. (C) IV = continuous intravenous infusion; (I) IV = intermittent intravenous infusion.
- Prepare a fresh infusion every 24 hours unless otherwise specified.
- Presume suitability as single-use only unless otherwise specified.
- Always check with additional reference sources regarding compatibility information – see Section A, 2.2.

Formulation	Method	Dilution	Rate	Comments	Compatibility
Ranitidine					
Ampoule 50 mg/2 mL	IV bolus	Dilute each 50 mg with a minimum of 20 mL N/S or G. Fluid restriction: undiluted (anecdotal).	Min. 2 minutes.	**Acute events that may accompany administration:** Rapid administration may occasionally produce bradycardia. **pH:** 6.7–7.3 **Flush:** N/S, G or G/S **Sodium content:** Negligible	**Y-site compatible (but see Section A, 2.6):** aciclovir, amikacin, aminophylline, atracurium, ceftazidime, ciprofloxacin, clarithromycin, dobutamine, dopamine, fentanyl, fluconazole, foscarnet, furosemide, glyceryl trinitrate, heparin, labetalol, midazolam, noradrenaline (norepinephrine), pancuronium, sodium bicarbonate.
	(I) IV infusion	Dilute to 100 mL with N/S or G.	25 mg/hour for 2 hours.		
	(C) IV infusion following initial IV bolus		150 micrograms/kg per hour.		
	Deep IM	Ready diluted.			

Formulation	Method	Dilution	Rate	Comments	Compatibility
Rasburicase					
Vials 1.5 mg or 7.5 mg	(I) IV infusion	Reconstitute with supplied solvent then dilute in 50 mL N/S.	30 minutes.	**Acute events that may accompany administration:** Allergic-type reactions, mainly rashes. Can cause hypotension, bronchospasm, rhinitis and severe hypersensitivity reactions including anaphylaxis. **pH:** 7.7–8.3 **Flush:** N/S **Sodium content:** 2 mmol/mL **Displacement:** Nil **Other Comments:** Do not shake the reconstituted vial. Rasburicase administered to patients with G-6-phosphate dehydrogenase (G6PD) deficiency can cause severe haemolysis.	Rasburicase solution should be infused through a different line from that used for infusion of chemotherapeutic agents to prevent any possible medicine incompatibility. If use of a separate line is not possible, the line should be flushed out with N/S solution between chemotherapeutic agent infusions and rasburicase. No filter should be used for infusion. **Incompatible:** G.

- For abbreviations used in the Table, see Section A, 2.4.
  e.g. (C) IV = continuous intravenous infusion; (I) IV = intermittent intravenous infusion.
- Prepare a fresh infusion every 24 hours unless otherwise specified.
- Presume suitability as single-use only unless otherwise specified.
- Always check with additional reference sources regarding compatibility information – see Section A, 2.2.

Formulation	Method	Dilution	Rate	Comments	Compatibility
Remifentanil					
Vial 1 mg, 2 mg, 5 mg	IV bolus	Reconstitute with N/S, G, or W to a concentration of 1 mg/mL then dilute further to a concentration of 20–250 micrograms/mL. (See below – (C) IV infusion).	See manufacturer's literature for dosing information	**Acute events that may accompany administration:** Muscle rigidity, marked respiratory depression, hypotension and bradycardia. **pH:** 2.5–3.5 **Flush:** Not recommended. Sufficient amount of remifentanil may be present in the dead space of the IV line and/or cannula. Inadvertent administration may be avoided by administering remifentanil into a fast-flowing IV line or via a dedicated IV line, which is removed when remifentanil is discontinued. **Sodium content:** Nil **Displacement:** Negligible **Other comments:** Administer only in a setting fully equipped for the monitoring and support of respiratory and cardiovascular function.	**Compatible** with the following when administered into a running IV catheter: alfentanil, adrenaline (epinephrine), aminophylline, calcium gluconate, ceftazidime, ceftriaxone, cefuroxime, dexamethasone, dobutamine, fentanyl, furosemide, granisetron, heparin sodium, hydrocortisone sodium succinate, lidocaine, lorazepam, magnesium, mannitol, methylprednisolone sodium succinate, metoclopramide, metronidazole, midazolam, morphine, noradrenaline (norepinephrine), phenylephrine, piperacillin, potassium chloride, prochlorperazine, propofol, theophylline, thiopental sodium.

Formulation	Method	Dilution	Rate	Comments	Compatibility
	(C) IV infusion	Reconstitute with N/S, G or W to a concentration of 1 mg/mL then dilute further to a concentration of 20–250 micrograms/mL. Local practice for adult general anaesthesia: 40 micrograms/mL (i.e. 2 mg in 50 mL).	See manu-facturer's literature for dosing information.		**Incompatible:** chlorpromazine, diazepam, amphoteracin B, pantoprazole.

- For abbreviations used in the Table, see Section A, 2.4.
  e.g. (C) IV = continuous intravenous infusion; (I) IV = intermittent intravenous infusion.
- Prepare a fresh infusion every 24 hours unless otherwise specified.
- Presume suitability as single-use only unless otherwise specified.
- Always check with additional reference sources regarding compatibility information – see Section A, 2.2.

Formulation	Method	Dilution	Rate	Comments	Compatibility
Rifampicin					
Vial 600mg	(I) IV infusion	Reconstitute with diluent provided and shake vigorously for 30–60 seconds then dilute with 500mL G (Rifadin).	2–3 hours.	**Acute events that may accompany administration:** May colour the urine, sputum and tears orange-red. Soft contact lens may be permanently discoloured and should not be worn during therapy. **pH:** 8–8.8 **Flush:** N/S **Sodium content:** <0.5mmol/600mg **Displacement:** Add 10mL diluent to 600mg vial to give a concentration of 60mg/1mL. Overage in vial will compensate for displacement volume. **Other comments:** Discard infusion after 6 hours.	Do not infuse with other medicines.
	(I) IV infusion for fluid restriction (unlicensed).	Reconstitute with diluent provided then dilute Rifadin 300–600mg in 100mL preferably with G, otherwise N/S.	2–3 hours.		

208

Formulation	Method	Dilution	Rate	Comments	Compatibility
Ritodrine					
Ampoule 50 mg/5 mL	(C) IV infusion via syringe pump (preferred method).	Dilute to 3 mg/1 mL with G.	Variable, see package insert. Max. rate 350 micrograms/minute.	**Acute events that may accompany administration:** Pulmonary oedema, monitor fluid balance and keep volume of infusion to a minimum. Tachycardia and palpitations – monitor maternal heart rate. Hypotension (left lateral position to minimise risk). Closely monitor blood glucose levels in patients with diabetes. **pH:** 4.8–5.5 **Flush:** G or N/S **Other comments:** The diluent should usually be G, but N/S can be used if clinically indicated, e.g. patient with diabetes.	
	(C) IV infusion without a syringe pump.	Dilute to 300 micrograms/1 mL with G.			
	IM	Ready diluted.			
Rocuronium					
Ampoule 50 mg/5 mL, 100 mg/10 mL	IV bolus	Ready diluted.	15–30 seconds.	**Acute events that may accompany administration:** High doses (greater than 0.9 mg/kg) may cause an increase in heart rate. **pH:** 4 **Flush:** G or N/S **Sodium content:** 1.5 mmol/50 mg	**Incompatible:** amoxicillin, amphoteracin, azathioprine, dexamethasone, erythromycin, furosemide, insulin (soluble), thiopentone, vancomycin.
	(C) IV infusion	May be diluted with N/S, G or G/S.	0.3–0.6 mg/kg per hour adjusted to response.		

- For abbreviations used in the Table, see Section A, 2.4.
  - e.g. (C) IV = continuous intravenous infusion; (I) IV = intermittent intravenous infusion.
- Prepare a fresh infusion every 24 hours unless otherwise specified.
- Presume suitability as single-use only unless otherwise specified.
- Always check with additional reference sources regarding compatibility information – see Section A, 2.2.

209

Formulation	Method	Dilution	Rate	Comments	Compatibility
Salbutamol					
Ampoule 500 micrograms/ 1 mL, 5 mg/5 mL for infusion	IV bolus	Dilute 500 micrograms/ 1 mL ampoule to 50 micrograms/ 1 mL with W.	3–5 minutes.	**Acute events that may accompany administration:** Increases in heart rate; monitor **ECG**. Rarely hypersensitivity reactions, including urticaria, bronchospasm and hypotension; monitor blood pressure. Extravasation may cause tissue damage; for management guidelines, see Section A, 7. **pH:** 3.5 **Flush:** N/S or G **Sodium content:** 0.15 mmol/1 mL **Other comments:** Salbutamol may be diluted with W, N/S or G. IM injection may produce slight pain or stinging.	**Incompatible:** aminophylline.
	(C) IV infusion for asthma.	Dilute to 10 micrograms/ 1 mL with G (i.e. 5 mL of 5 mg/5 mL added to 495 mL of G). Fluid restricted: 10 mg in 50 mL (anecdotal).			

Formulation	Method	Dilution	Rate	Comments	Compatibility
	(C) IV infusion for premature labour via syringe pump.	Dilute to 200 micrograms/1mL with G (i.e. 10mL of 5mg/5mL added to 40mL of G).			
	(C) IV infusion for premature labour if syringe pump is unavailable.	Dilute to 20 micrograms/1mL with G (i.e. 10mL of 5mg/5mL added to 490mL of G).			
	IM or S/C.	Ready diluted.			

- For abbreviations used in the Table, see Section A, 2.4.
  e.g. (C) IV = continuous intravenous infusion; (I) IV = intermittent intravenous infusion.
- Prepare a fresh infusion every 24 hours unless otherwise specified.
- Presume suitability as single-use only unless otherwise specified.
- Always check with additional reference sources regarding compatibility information – see Section A, 2.2.

Formulation	Method	Dilution	Rate	Comments	Compatibility
Sodium benzoate (unlicensed)					
Ampoule 1 g/5 mL, 5 g/25 mL	(I) or (C) IV infusion	Seek specialist advice. Add dose to 100 mL G (local practice) or N/S.		**Acute events that may accompany administration:** Vomiting. **Sodium content:** 3.5 mmol/500 mg	

Formulation	Method	Dilution	Rate	Comments	Compatibility
Sodium bicarbonate					
Infusion bag 1.26% 500mL, Polyfusor 4.2% 500mL, Infusion bottle 8.4% 100mL, Ampoule 4.2% 10mL, 8.4% 10mL, Ampoule 1% 2mL, 5mL	(C) IV infusion	Use ready-prepared infusions when possible. May be diluted with N/S or G.	Variable.	**Acute events that may accompany administration:** Extravasation may cause tissue damage; for management guidelines, see Section A, 7. **pH:** 7–8.5 **Flush:** N/S or G **Other comments:** Concentrations >1.26% should be given via a central line. For prevention of contrast media-induced nephropathy: (C) IV infusion of 1.26% at 3mL/kg per hour for 1 hour pre-contrast followed by 1mL/kg per hour for 6 hour post-contrast. If weight >110kg, use 110kg to calculate dose.	**Y-site compatible (but see Section A, 2.6):** aciclovir, dexamethasone, fentanyl, heparin sodium, potassium chloride, piperacillin/tazobactam, propofol, vancomycin. **Incompatible:** amiodarone, ceftazidime, ciprofloxacin, cisplatin, dobutamine, dopamine, imipenem/cilastin, insulin (soluble), labetalol, midazolam, morphine, ondansetron noradrenaline (norepinephrine), solutions containing calcium, magnesium or phosphate.
	IV bolus	Ready diluted.			
	(I) IV infusion	Use ready-prepared infusions when possible. May be diluted with N/S or G.	Variable.		

- For abbreviations used in the Table, see Section A, 2.4.
  e.g. (C) IV = continuous intravenous infusion; (I) IV = intermittent intravenous infusion.
- Prepare a fresh infusion every 24hours unless otherwise specified.
- Presume suitability as single-use only unless otherwise specified.
- Always check with additional reference sources regarding compatibility information – see Section A, 2.2.

213

Formulation	Method	Dilution	Rate	Comments	Compatibility
Sodium calcium edetate					
Ampoule 1000 mg/5 mL	(I) IV infusion via volumetric infusion pump.	Dilute with 250–500 mL N/S or G (max. concentration 3% [3000 mg/100 mL]).	Min. 1 hour	**Acute events that may accompany administration:** Thrombophlebitis if given too rapidly. **pH:** 6.5–8 **Flush:** N/S, G **Sodium content:** 5.3 mmol/1000 mg **Other comments:** IM injection is painful, add a local anaesthetic.	Do not infuse with other medicines.
	IM (unlicensed) See 'Other comments'.	Ready diluted.			
	S/C (unlicensed)				

Formulation	Method	Dilution	Rate	Comments	Compatibility
Sodium chloride					
Ampoule 0.9% 2mL, 5mL, 10mL. 30%, 10mL. Infusion bags 0.9% 100mL, 250mL, 500mL, 1000mL. 0.45%, 1.8%, 2.7%, 5% 500mL	(C) or (I) IV infusion	Use ready-prepared infusions when possible.		**Acute events that may accompany administration:** Vein irritation with concentrated solutions. **pH:** 4.5–7 **Sodium content:** 150mmol/1L (0.9% injection). **Other comments:** Concentrations >1.8% should be given via a central line.	Check under individual medicine monograph.
	IV bolus	Concentrated solutions may be diluted with N/S, G, G/S or H.			

- For abbreviations used in the Table, see Section A, 2.4.
  e.g. (C) IV = continuous intravenous infusion; (I) IV = intermittent intravenous infusion.
- Prepare a fresh infusion every 24 hours unless otherwise specified.
- Presume suitability as single-use only unless otherwise specified.
- Always check with additional reference sources regarding compatibility information – see Section A, 2.2.

215

Formulation	Method	Dilution	Rate	Comments	Compatibility
Sodium fusidate					
Vial 500mg	(I) IV infusion into a central venous line (preferred method).	Reconstitute with 10mL buffered diluent provided then dilute with at least 500mL N/S, G or G/S.	2 hours.	**Acute events that may accompany administration:** Pain at injection site. Rapid infusion may cause venospasm, haemolysis of erythrocytes and thrombophlebitis. **pH:** 7.4–7.6 after reconstitution with buffer. **Flush:** N/S **Sodium and phosphate content:** When reconstituted with 10mL buffer contains 3.1mmol sodium and 1.1mmol phosphate. **Displacement:** Negligible **Other comments:** G or G/S can be used as diluent but opalescence may occur with more acidic samples. Infusion must be discarded if this occurs.	**Incompatible:** G infusions of 20% and above. Precipitation may occur with solutions of pH < 7.4.
		Fluid restricted: centrally 500mg in 100mL, peripherally 500mg in 250mL (anecdotal).	Minimum 6 hours.		
	(I) IV infusion into large peripheral vein.	As above.	Minimum 6 hours.		

Formulation	Method	Dilution	Rate	Comments	Compatibility
Sodium nitroprusside					
Vial 50 mg	(C) IV infusion via syringe or volumetric infusion pump.	ITU local practice: reconstitute vial with 2 mL G provided, then further dilute to 50 mg/50 mL in G or N/S (dilution with N/S is unlicensed). Alternatively, reconstitute vial with 2 mL G provided, then further dilute in 250–1000 mL G (max. concentration of 200 micrograms/1 mL). This is the licensed recommendation.	Increase rate slowly until desired effect occurs. Discontinue infusion gradually over 10–30 minutes.	**Acute events that may accompany administration: Hypotension;** monitor blood pressure. Rapid reduction in blood pressure can lead to nausea, vomiting, headache and abdominal pain. These effects can be reduced by slowing infusion rate. Side effects caused by excessive plasma concentration of the cyanide metabolite include tachycardia, sweating, hyperventilation, arrhythmias, and marked metabolic acidosis. Extravasation may cause tissue damage; for management guidelines, see Section A, 7. **pH:** 3.5–6 (in G) **Do not flush:** Replace giving set **Sodium content:** 0.34 mmol/50 mg **Displacement:** Negligible **Other comments:** Protect infusion from light (wrap infusion solution and tubing in aluminium foil). A faint brown tint in the infusion solution is normal. Do not use if highly coloured. If more than 3 days therapy, monitor blood thiocyanate levels.	**Y-site compatible (but see Section A, 2.6):** atracurium, dopamine, dobutamine (both medicines in N/S), glyceryl trinitrate, heparin sodium, insulin (soluble), labetolol, lidocaine, midazolam, morphine, pancuronium, propofol, vecuronium. **Incompatible:** haloperidol, levofloxacin.

- For abbreviations used in the Table, see Section A, 2.4.
- e.g. (C) IV = continuous intravenous infusion; (I) IV = intermittent intravenous infusion.
- Prepare a fresh infusion every 24 hours unless otherwise specified.
- Presume suitability as single-use only unless otherwise specified.
- Always check with additional reference sources regarding compatibility information – see Section A, 2.2.

Formulation	Method	Dilution	Rate	Comments	Compatibility
Sodium phenylbutyrate (unlicensed)					
Vial 1 g/5 mL	(I) or (C) IV infusion	Seek specialist advice.		**Acute events that may accompany administration:** Nausea, vomiting, irritability. **Sodium content:** 2.7 mmol/500 mg	

Formulation	Method	Dilution	Rate	Comments	Compatibility
Sodium stibogluconate					
Vial 100mL, equivalent to 100mg/1mL pentavalent antimony	IV bolus	Ready diluted. Draw up dose through a 5 μm filter. Do not administer through filter (local practice).	5 minutes.	**Acute events that may accompany administration:** Rapid administration may cause local thrombosis. If coughing, vomiting or substernal pain occurs, discontinue administration. **ECG** monitoring is necessary in heart disease. **pH:** 5.6 **Flush:** W **Other comments:** The contents of vial can be used for up to 48 hours (local practice). Return to pharmacy for disposal. IM injection is painful.	
	(I) IV infusion (unlicensed)	Draw up dose through a 5 μm filter. Dilute dose in 100mL N/S. Do not administer through filter (local practice).	30 minutes.		
	IM injection	Ready diluted.			

- For abbreviations used in the Table, see Section A, 2.4.
  e.g. (C) IV = continuous intravenous infusion; (I) IV = intermittent intravenous infusion.
- Prepare a fresh infusion every 24hours unless otherwise specified.
- Presume suitability as single-use only unless otherwise specified.
- Always check with additional reference sources regarding compatibility information – see Section A, 2.2.

219

Formulation	Method	Dilution	Rate	Comments	Compatibility
Sodium valproate					
Vial 400 mg	IV bolus	Reconstitute with 4 mL diluent provided. Due to displacement the resulting concentration is 95 mg/1 mL. May be diluted with N/S, G or G/S.	3–5 minutes.	**Acute events that may accompany administration:** Vomiting, ataxia, jaundice, CNS depression – discontinue if these occur (may be sign of hepatic failure). **pH:** 6.8–8.5 **Flush:** N/S, G or G/S **Sodium content:** 2.41 mmol/400 mg vial.	Do not infuse with other medicines.
	(C) or (I) IV infusion via a syringe or volumetric infusion pump.	As above.			

Formulation	Method	Dilution	Rate	Comments	Compatibility
Sotalol					
Ampoule 40 mg/4 mL	IV bolus	Ready diluted.	Minimum 10 minutes.	**Acute events that may accompany administration:** Bradycardia and hypotension, monitor **ECG** and blood pressure. **pH:** 4.3–5.2 **Flush:** N/S, G **Sodium content:** 0.5 mmol/ampoule	
	(C) or (I) IV infusion	Dilute to a concentration of between 10 and 2000 micrograms/mL with either N/S or G.	See manufacturer's literature		

- For abbreviations used in the Table, see Section A, 2.4.
  e.g. (C) IV = continuous intravenous infusion; (I) IV = intermittent intravenous infusion.
- Prepare a fresh infusion every 24 hours unless otherwise specified.
- Presume suitability as single-use only unless otherwise specified.
- Always check with additional reference sources regarding compatibility information – see Section A, 2.2.

Formulation	Method	Dilution	Rate	Comments	Compatibility
Streptokinase					
Vial 250000 units, 750000 units, 1500000 units	(C) or (I) IV infusion via volumetric infusion or syringe pump.	Streptase brand: reconstitute all sizes with 5mL N/S.	Dependent on indication; see package insert for details.	**Acute events that may accompany administration:** Hypotension and arrhythmias, monitor blood pressure and **ECG**. Fever, haemorrhage, chills and major allergic reactions. **pH:** 6.8–7.5 **Flush:** N/S **Displacement:** None **Other comments:** Discard infusion after 12 hours.	**Y-site compatible (but see Section A, 2.6):** amiodarone, digoxin, dobutamine, dopamine, flecainide, glyceryl trinitrate, heparin, insulin (soluble), lidocaine, magnesium sulphate.
Sulfadiazine					
Ampoule 1g/4mL	(I) IV infusion (preferred method).	Dilute dose with N/S to a maximum concentration of 50mg/1mL. Preferably dilute required dose in 500mL to 1L N/S to reduce risk of crystallisation of sulfadiazine in the urine.	Minimum 30–60 minutes.	**Acute events that may accompany administration:** Risk of crystallisation in the urine. A high fluid intake (2.5–3.5L in 24 hours) should be maintained and urine output should not be less than half that amount. Nausea; give regular antiemetics half an hour before infusion starts. Extravasation may cause tissue damage; for management guidelines, see Section A, 7. **pH:** 11 (approximately) **Flush:** N/S **Sodium content:** Approximately 4mmol/1g	**Incompatible:** acids, aminoglycosides, iron salts and salts of heavy metals, G, hydralazine, insulin (soluble), noradrenaline (norepinephrine).
	Deep IM	Ready diluted.			

Formulation	Method	Dilution	Rate	Comments	Compatibility
Suxamethonium					
Ampoule 100 mg/2 mL	IV bolus	Ready diluted.	10–30 seconds.	**Acute events that may accompany administration:** Prolonged neuromuscular blockade, bradycardia, hyper-and hypotension, muscle pain, anaphylaxis. **pH:** 3–4.5 **Flush:** N/S or G **Sodium content:** Negligible	**Y-site compatible (but see Section A, 2.6):** heparin, morphine, potassium chloride, propofol. **Incompatible:** do not mix with anything else in same syringe. Generally incompatible with alkaline solutions, e.g. thiopental.
	(C) IV infusion via volumetric infusion or syringe pump.	Dilute to 1–2 mg/1 mL with G, N/S or G/S.	2–4 mg/minute		
	IM	Ready diluted.			

- For abbreviations used in the Table, see Section A, 2.4.
- e.g. (C) IV = continuous intravenous infusion; (I) IV = intermittent intravenous infusion.
- Prepare a fresh infusion every 24 hours unless otherwise specified.
- Presume suitability as single-use only unless otherwise specified.
- Always check with additional reference sources regarding compatibility information – see Section A, 2.2.

223

Formulation	Method	Dilution	Rate	Comments	Compatibility
Tacrolimus					
Ampoule 5 mg/mL (1 mL ampoule)	(C) IV infusion	Dilute required dose from the concentrate in N/S or G to a final concentration of 0.004–0.1 mg/mL (4–100 micrograms/ mL). Total fluid volume of infusion over 24 hours should be in the range 20–250 mL. Do not give as a bolus.		**Acute events that may accompany administration:** Infusion solution contains polyoxyethylene hydrogenated castor oil, which has been reported to cause anaphylactoid reactions. **Flush:** N/S or G **Sodium content:** Negligible **Displacement:** N/A **Other comments:** The content of the concentrate for infusion is not compatible with PVC. Tubing, syringes and any other equipment used to administer tacrolimus should not contain PVC. Infusion solution contains ethanol (638 mg/mL).	Tacrolimus is not compatible with PVC plastics. Avoid mixing tacrolimus with other medicines. In particular mixed infusions with medicines that are alkaline in solution (e.g. aciclovir, ganciclovir) must not be administered because tacrolimus can degrade under these conditions.

224

Formulation	Method	Dilution	Rate	Comments	Compatibility
Teicoplanin					
Vial 200 mg, 400 mg	IV bolus	Add W provided to vial and roll gently until completely reconstituted, taking care to avoid formation of foam. If foam is formed then allow to stand for 15 minutes for foam to subside. May be further diluted with N/S, G or G/S.	3–5 minutes.	**pH:** 7.5 **Flush:** N/S, G **Sodium content:** <0.5 mmol/vial (200 mg and 400 mg). **Displacement:** 0.59 mL/1 g. Manufacturer allows for displacement; when reconstituted as directed 200 mg vial contains 200 mg/3 mL and 400 mg vial contains 400 mg/3 mL.	**Incompatible:** aminoglycosides.
	(I) IV infusion	As above.	30 minutes.		
	IM	Reconstitute as described for 'IV bolus'.			

- For abbreviations used in the Table, see Section A, 2.4.
  e.g. (C) IV = continuous intravenous infusion; (I) IV = intermittent intravenous infusion.
- Prepare a fresh infusion every 24 hours unless otherwise specified.
- Presume suitability as single-use only unless otherwise specified.
- Always check with additional reference sources regarding compatibility information – see Section A, 2.2.

225

Formulation	Method	Dilution	Rate	Comments	Compatibility
Terbutaline					
Ampoule 500 micrograms/ 1 mL, 2.5 mg/5 mL for infusion	IV bolus	May be diluted with N/S or G.	Minimum 3–5 minutes.	**Acute events that may accompany administration:** Tremor, palpitations, dizziness and nervousness. Monitor blood pressure, heart rate and blood glucose in patients with diabetes. Pain at injection site may occur with S/C administration. Maternal pulmonary oedema; monitor hydration status of patient. Extravasation may cause tissue damage; for management guidelines, see Section A, 7. **pH:** 3–5 **Flush:** N/S or G	**Y-site compatible (but see Section A, 2.6):** aminophylline, doxapram, insulin (soluble).
	(C) IV infusion for bronchodilation	Dilute 3 mL (1.5 mg) of the 2.5 mg/5 mL ampoule or 5 mL (2.5 mg) with 500 mL N/S, G or G/S to give a concentration of 3 micrograms/ 1 mL or 5 micrograms/ 1 mL.	**Adults:** 1.5–5 micrograms/ minute for 8–10 hours.	**Sodium content:** 0.15 mmol/1 mL **Other comments:** IM and S/C injections are preferred to IV bolus for bronchodilation. In order to minimise the risk of hypotension associated with tocolytic therapy, special care should be taken to avoid caval compression by keeping the patient in the left or right lateral positions throughout the infusion.	

Formulation	Method	Dilution	Rate	Comments	Compatibility
	(C) IV infusion for pre-term labour via syringe pump.	Dilute 10 mL (5 mg) of the 2.5 mg/5 mL ampoule with 40 mL G to produce a 100 micrograms/ 1 mL solution.	See package insert.		
	(C) IV infusion for pre-term labour via volumetric infusion pump.	Dilute 10 mL (5 mg of the 2.5 mg/5 mL ampoule) with 490 mL G to produce a 10 micrograms/ 1 mL solution.	See package insert.		
	IM or S/C	Ready diluted.			
	(C) S/C infusion via syringe pump for patients with brittle asthma (unlicensed).	Ready diluted.	See specialist guidelines for details.		

- For abbreviations used in the Table, see Section A, 2.4.
  e.g. (C) IV = continuous intravenous infusion; (I) IV = intermittent intravenous infusion.
- Prepare a fresh infusion every 24 hours unless otherwise specified.
- Presume suitability as single-use only unless otherwise specified.
- Always check with additional reference sources regarding compatibility information – see Section A, 2.2.

227

Formulation	Method	Dilution	Rate	Comments	Compatibility
Terlipressin acetate					
1 mg vial/5 mL solvent included	IV bolus	Reconstitute each 1 mg vial with the solvent provided (5 mL).	3–4 minutes.	**Acute events that may accompany administration:** Hypertension, cardiac dysrhythmias, electrolyte disturbances. **Flush:** N/S **Sodium content:** solvent only – N/S (approx. 5 mL). **Displacement:** After reconstitution – final volume 5.2–5.5 mL (varies with solvent). **Other comments:** Keep the container in the outer carton. After reconstitution with the solvent provided, vials should be used immediately.	
Tetracosactide (tetracosactrin)					
Ampoule 250 micrograms/ 1 mL	IV bolus	Ready diluted.	2 minutes.	**Acute events that may accompany administration:** Hypersensitivity reactions, anaphylactic shock in patients with allergic disorders. Extravasation may cause tissue damage; for management guidelines, see Section A, 7. **pH:** 3.8–4.5 **Flush:** N/S, G **Sodium content:** Negligible	
	IM	Ready diluted.			

228

Formulation	Method	Dilution	Rate	Comments	Compatibility
Thiopental (thiopentone)					
Ampoule 500mg, Vial 2.5g	IV bolus	Reconstitute 500mg with 20mL W or 2.5g in 100mL W to produce a 2.5% solution. The dose may be further diluted with N/S or G (unlicensed diluent).	10–15 seconds.	**Acute events that may accompany administration:** Hypotension; monitor blood pressure, hypersensitivity reactions. Extravasation may cause tissue damage. Treat extravasation by immediate infiltration of hyaluronidase in a local anaesthetic; for general extravasation treatment guidelines, see Section A, 7. **pH:** 10.5 (2.5% solution) **Flush:** N/S **Other comments:** Check for haze or precipitation before administering. Solutions decompose on standing. Solutions should be freshly prepared, stored at 2–8°C and used within 7 hours. **Sodium content:** 4.9 mmol/1 g.	Do not infuse with other medicines.
	(I) IV infusion	Reconstitute as above then dilute to 0.2–0.4% (2–4mg/1mL) with N/S or G (unlicensed diluent).			
	(C) IV infusion (unlicensed)	As for (I) IV infusion.			

- For abbreviations used in the Table, see Section A, 2.4.
  e.g. (C) IV = continuous intravenous infusion; (I) IV = intermittent intravenous infusion.
- Prepare a fresh infusion every 24 hours unless otherwise specified.
- Presume suitability as single-use only unless otherwise specified.
- Always check with additional reference sources regarding compatibility information – see Section A, 2.2.

Formulation	Method	Dilution	Rate	Comments	Compatibility
Tobramycin					
Vial 20mg/2mL, 40mg/1mL, 80mg/2mL	(I) IV infusion (preferred method).	Dilute required dose in 50–100mL N/S or G.	20–60 minutes.	**Acute events that may accompany administration:** Allergic type reactions including anaphylaxis to the preservative sodium bisulphite. Extravasation may cause tissue damage; for management guidelines, see Section A, 7. **pH:** 3.5–6 **Flush:** N/S or G **Other comments:** Plasma level monitoring is required.	**Y-site compatible (but see Section A, 2.6):** aciclovir (both medicines in G), ciprofloxacin, metronidazole. **Incompatible:** amoxicillin, cefotaxime, ceftazidime, cefuroxime, co-amoxiclav, flucloxacillin, heparin, teicoplanin, trimethoprim.
	IV bolus	May be diluted with N/S or G.	3–5 minutes.		
	IM	Ready diluted.			

Formulation	Method	Dilution	Rate	Comments	Compatibility
Tramadol					
Ampoule 100 mg/2 mL	IV bolus	Ready diluted.	2–3 minutes.	**Acute events that may accompany administration:** Rapid intravenous administration associated with a higher incidence of adverse effects. Nausea, vomiting, skin rashes. Monitor for typical symptoms of opioid analgesic overdose. Treat with supportive measures and naloxone to reverse respiratory depression. **pH:** 6–6.8 **Flush:** N/S **Sodium content:** Negligible	**Incompatible:** diazepam, diclofenac, indometacin, midazolam.
	(I) or (C) IV infusion	Dilute dose to a convenient volume in N/S, G, H, or G/S.			
	IM	Ready diluted.			

- For abbreviations used in the Table, see Section A, 2.4.
  e.g. (C) IV = continuous intravenous infusion; (I) IV = intermittent intravenous infusion.
- Prepare a fresh infusion every 24 hours unless otherwise specified.
- Presume suitability as single-use only unless otherwise specified.
- Always check with additional reference sources regarding compatibility information – see Section A, 2.2.

Formulation	Method	Dilution	Rate	Comments	Compatibility
Tranexamic acid					
Ampoule 500mg/5mL	IV bolus (preferred method)	May be diluted with N/S or G.	100mg/minute.	**Acute events that may accompany administration:** Rapid injection may cause dizziness and/or hypotension. **pH:** 6.5–8 **Flush:** N/S or G **Sodium content:** Nil	**Y-site compatible (but see Section A, 2.6):** heparin **Incompatible:** penicillins
	(C) IV infusion	As above.	25–50mg/kg per 24 hours.		

Formulation	Method	Dilution	Rate	Comments	Compatibility
TRH					
	See Protirelin				
Urokinase (unlicensed)					
Vial 5000 units, 25000 units, 100000 units	IV bolus to unblock 'AV' shunts and IV cannulae.	Reconstitute 5000–25000 units with 2–3mL N/S. To unblock haemodialysis lines, Permacaths, shunts and Hickman lines: leave to dwell in affected lumen for at least 1 hour and preferably 2–4 hours. Remove lysate and flush.		**pH:** 5.5–7 **Flush:** N/S **Sodium content:** Negligible	

- For abbreviations used in the Table, see Section A, 2.4.
  e.g. (C) IV = continuous intravenous infusion; (I) IV = intermittent intravenous infusion.
- Prepare a fresh infusion every 24hours unless otherwise specified.
- Presume suitability as single-use only unless otherwise specified.
- Always check with additional reference sources regarding compatibility information – see Section A, 2.2.

233

Formulation	Method	Dilution	Rate	Comments	Compatibility
Vancomycin					
Vial 500 mg, 1 g	(I) IV infusion	Reconstitute each 500 mg with 10 mL W, then dilute with a minimum of 100 mL N/S or G. Fluid restriction: 1 g in 100 mL via a fast-flowing vein (unlicensed).	Minimum 60 minutes (max. rate 10 mg/minute).	**Acute events that may accompany administration:** Anaphylactoid reactions including hypotension, wheezing, dyspnoea, urticaria or pruritus. Rapid infusion may cause flushing of the upper body ('red neck') or pain and muscle spasm of the chest and back. Extravasation may cause tissue damage; for management guidelines, see Section A, 7. **pH:** 2.8–4.5 **Flush:** N/S or G **Displacement:** 0.3 mL/500 mg vial Add 9.7 mL W to 500 mg vial to give a concentration of 50 mg/1 mL.	**Y-site compatible (but see Section A, 2.6):** aciclovir, amiodarone, atracurium, clarithromycin, fluconazole, meropenem, midazolam, morphine, ondansetron. **Incompatible:** barbiturates, ceftazidime, cefotaxime, ceftriaxone, cefuroxime, dexamethasone, foscarnet, heparin, omeprazole, piperacillin/tazobactam.
	(C) IV infusion (unlicensed practice in some centres).	As above.			

Formulation	Method	Dilution	Rate	Comments	Compatibility
Vecuronium					
Vial 10 mg	IV bolus	Reconstitute with 5 mL W (diluent provided). May be diluted to 1 mg/1 mL with W, N/S, G, G/S or Ringer's.	Rapidly.	**Acute events that may accompany administration:** Erythematous reactions at injection site. **pH:** 4 **Flush:** N/S or G	**Y-site compatible (but see Section A, 2.6):** aminophylline, cefuroxime, clarithromycin, dobutamine, dopamine, fentanyl, fluconazole, gentamicin, glyceryl trinitrate, heparin sodium, labetalol, lorazepam, midazolam, morphine, noradrenaline (norepinephrine), propofol, sodium nitroprusside, vancomycin. **Incompatible:** etomidate, furosemide, thiopental and other alkaline agents.
	(C) IV infusion	Reconstitute with 5 mL W (diluent provided). Dilute with N/S or G to a maximum concentration of 4 mg/100 mL.			

- For abbreviations used in the Table, see Section A, 2.4.
  e.g. (C) IV = continuous intravenous infusion; (I) IV = intermittent intravenous infusion.
- Prepare a fresh infusion every 24 hours unless otherwise specified.
- Presume suitability as single-use only unless otherwise specified.
- Always check with additional reference sources regarding compatibility information – see Section A, 2.2.

235

Formulation	Method	Dilution	Rate	Comments	Compatibility
Verapamil					
Ampoule 5 mg/2 mL	IV bolus	May be diluted with N/S or G.	2 minutes (3 minutes in elderly people).	**Acute events that may accompany administration:** Reduced heart rate, transient hypotension, monitor blood pressure and **ECG**. Reduced contractility and in extreme cases asystole. Rarely flushing, headache, vertigo, allergic reactions. **pH:** 4–6.5 **Flush:** N/S, G **Sodium content:** 0.3 mmol/ampoule.	**Y-site compatible (but see Section A, 2.6):** amiodarone, atropine, bretylium, calcium salts, digoxin, dopamine, furosemide, glyceryl trinitrate, heparin, insulin (soluble), magnesium sulphate, potassium chloride, sodium bicarbonate. **Incompatible:** hydralazine, alkaline solutions.

Formulation	Method	Dilution	Rate	Comments	Compatibility
Vitamins B and C					
	See Pabrinex IVHP				
Vitamin K					
	See Phyto-menadione				

- For abbreviations used in the Table, see Section A, 2.4.
  e.g. (C) IV = continuous intravenous infusion; (I) IV = intermittent intravenous infusion.
- Prepare a fresh infusion every 24 hours unless otherwise specified.
- Presume suitability as single-use only unless otherwise specified.
- Always check with additional reference sources regarding compatibility information – see Section A, 2.2.

Formulation	Method	Dilution	Rate	Comments	Compatibility
Voriconazole					
Vial 200 mg	(I) IV infusion	Reconstitute 200 mg vial with 19 mL W, giving a concentration of 10 mg/mL. Discard vial if vacuum does not pull diluent into vial. Dilute dose in N/S or G to a final concentration of 0.5–5 mg/mL.	60–120 minutes. Max. rate 3 mg/kg per hour	**Acute events that may accompany administration:** Infusion-related reactions, predominantly flushing and nausea, have been observed during administration. Depending on the severity of symptoms, consideration should be given to stopping treatment. **pH:** 5.5–7.5 **Flush:** N/S or G **Sodium content:** 9.62 mmol/200 mg vial **Displacement:** Reconstitute 200 mg vial with 19 mL W to give 200 mg/20 mL. **Other comments:** Risk of accumulation of excipient (sulphobutylether β cyclodextrin sodium) in renal failure. Patients with renal impairment defined as creatinine clearance <50 mL/minute should not be treated with intravenous voriconazole.	Voriconazole must not be infused into the same line or cannula concomitantly with infusions of other medicinal products, including parenteral nutrition; 4.2% sodium bicarbonate is not compatible with voriconazole and is not recommended for use as a diluent. Infusions of blood products must not occur simultaneously with voriconazole.

238

Formulation	Method	Dilution	Rate	Comments	Compatibility
Zidovudine					
Vial 200mg/20mL	(C) IV infusion during labour (start infusion 4 hours before elective caesarean section).	Dilute to 2mg/1mL or 4mg/1mL with G. May be diluted with N/S if clinically indicated.	2mg/kg over 1 hour then 1mg/kg per hour until the umbilical cord is clamped	**Acute events that may accompany administration:** May cause pain, irritation and phlebitis at injection site. **pH:** 5.5 **Flush:** N/S or G	**Y-site compatible (but see Section A, 2.6):** aciclovir, co-trimoxazole. dexamethasone, fluconazole, heparin sodium, morphine, ondansetron, pentamidine, potassium chloride, clindamycin (both medicines in G).
	(I) IV infusion for patients temporarily NBM.	As above.	>60 minutes		

- For abbreviations used in the Table, see Section A, 2.4.
  e.g. (C) IV = continuous intravenous infusion; (I) IV = intermittent intravenous infusion.
- Prepare a fresh infusion every 24 hours unless otherwise specified.
- Presume suitability as single-use only unless otherwise specified.
- Always check with additional reference sources regarding compatibility information – see Section A, 2.2.

239